CONTROL DIABETES
IN SIX EASY STEPS

ALSO BY MAGGIE GREENWOOD-ROBINSON

Wrinkle-Free: Your Guide to Youthful Skin at Any Age

The Bone Density Test

The Cellulite Breakthrough

Hair Savers for Women: A Complete Guide to Treating and Preventing Hair Loss

Natural Weight Loss Miracles

21 Days to Better Fitness

Kava: The Ultimate Guide to Nature's Anti-Stress Herb

CONTROL DIABETES

IN SIX EASY STEPS

Maggie Greenwood-Robinson, Ph.D.

A LYNN SONBERG BOOK

St. Martin's Griffin
New York

CONTROL DIABETES IN SIX EASY STEPS. Copyright © 2002 by Lynn Sonberg. All rights reserved. Printed in the United States of America. For information, address St. Martin's Press, 175 Fifth Avenue, New York, N.Y. 10010.

www.stmartins.com

The author is grateful for permission to use commentary from the following individuals in sections of this book: Sherrye Landrum, associate director, Consumer Books, American Diabetes Association, for "Top-Ten Strategies for Learning About Your Diabetes"; Lori Bender, M.S., R.D., C.D.E., for "Top-Ten Strategies for Eating a Healthy, Healing Diet"; Kathleen Head, N.D., for "Top-Ten Strategies for Using Natural Remedies"; Sheri Colberg, Ph.D., for "Top-Ten Strategies for Exercise"; Richard P. Huemer, M.D., and Mary K. Michelis, M.D., for "Top-Ten Strategies for Getting the Best Possible Medical Care"; Judith Schwambach, Ph.D., for "Top-Ten Strategies for Emotional Well-Being."

Library of Congress Cataloging-in-Publication Data

Greenwood-Robinson, Maggie.
    Control diabetes in six easy steps / Maggie Greenwood-Robinson.
       p. cm.
    Includes bibliographical references and index.
    ISBN 0-312-28626-0
    1. Diabetes—Popular works. I. Title.

RC660.4 .G74 2002
616.4'62—dc21   2001058898

D 12 11 10 9 8 7

Important Note to the Reader

This book is for informational purposes only. It is not intended to take the place of medical advice from a trained medical professional. Readers are advised to consult a physician or other qualified health professional regarding treatment of all of their health problems or before acting on any of the information or advice in this book.

This book is intended to provide selected information about diabetes. Research about this complex condition is ongoing and subject to conflicting interpretations. As a result, there is no guarantee that what we know about this subject won't change with time.

Contents

Acknowledgments	ix
Author's Note	xi
Introduction: Embracing a New Way of Life	xiii

PART ONE: *Diabetes: What You Need to Know*

· Stopping a Silent Killer	3
· Unmasking Trouble: How Your Doctor Diagnoses Diabetes	24
· Preventing Life-Threatening Complications	28
· Choosing Quality Caregivers	38
· Medical Tests and Medications That Can Save Your Life	44
· Eat to Beat Diabetes: Understanding the Role of Nutrition	61
· The Exercise Connection	72

PART TWO: *Control Diabetes in Six Easy Steps*

- Step 1: Follow a Healing, Healthy Diet — *81*
- Step 2: Drive Diabetes into Retreat with Natural Remedies — *112*
- Step 3: Test Your Blood Sugar Regularly — *153*
- Step 4: Get Fit to Fight Diabetes — *163*
- Step 5: Take Medicine if Your Doctor Prescribes It — *187*
- Step 6: Defeat Stress with Positive Living — *207*

Glossary — *225*
Resources — *233*
References — *243*
Index — *257*

Acknowledgments

I gratefully thank the following people for their work and contributions to this book: my agent, Madeleine Morel, 2M Communications, Ltd.; Lynn Sonberg of Lynn Sonberg Book Associates; Richard P. Huemer, M.D.; Mary K. Michelis, M.D.; Sherrye Landrum of the American Diabetes Association; Lori Bender, M.S., R.D., C.D.E.; Kathleen Head, N.D.; Sheri Colberg, Ph.D.; and Judith Schwambach, Ph.D. I extend an additional thanks to Dr. Huemer for reviewing parts of the manuscript relating to medical care for people with diabetes.

Author's Note

Diabetes is a serious, potentially life-threatening disease. The suggestions and information presented in this book are not meant to substitute for regular, continuing medical care by a physician and other health care professionals. People with diabetes and their families are advised to consult a physician or other health care professional before undertaking any diet, supplementation, exercise, or medication program referred to in this book.

All questions and concerns regarding your diabetes and other medical conditions should be directed toward your physician.

Use of nutritional supplements, diabetes products, or medications is not recommended unless it is done under the guidance and supervision of a physician.

The mention of specific products or brands in this book does not constitute an endorsement by either the author or the publisher. The author has no financial interest in any companies that produce or market diabetes products or treatments. The information presented in this book was written solely on the merits of those products and treatments.

INTRODUCTION

Embracing a New Way of Life

You've probably heard the word *diabetes* for years without giving it much thought. Then, after a routine exam, your doctor tells you that you have it. The news may stop you cold. Naturally, it's upsetting to find out that you have a chronic disease and, just naturally, you may ask yourself, "Why me?"

At first, you may deny the diagnosis, thinking there has been some mistake. Denial is understandable, since it helps us cope initially with bad news. After the diagnosis sinks in, you may feel angry, depressed, worried, or overwhelmed with what it all means. You're frightened too, frightened of possibly having to depend on drugs for the rest of your life, of losing your independence, of complications, of being sick.

Your emotions are running high. But take heart: Such feelings are a perfectly normal part of the process that helps you come to terms with the fact that you have diabetes. Those same emotions will motivate you to take action and embrace a new way of life. If you don't and continue to ignore your diabetes, you're likely to develop the serious complications you fear most.

The good news—no, the great news—is that taking action to

control your diabetes is not as difficult as you might think. Yes, you have to alter some lifestyle habits, mostly involving healthier nutrition and increased physical activity. But the call to eat better and exercise more is no less than what every person on this planet needs to do—diabetes or no diabetes—to improve his or her health and find greater happiness. In other words, the lifestyle changes recommended for people with diabetes are the same ones recommended for your best friend, your coworkers, your next-door neighbor, and every member of your family. In some ways, you're luckier than they are. You now have a stronger-than-ever impetus to make some health-enhancing changes in your lifestyle.

Once you start making these changes, some rather remarkable things will take place in your life. You'll look better, feel better, and have more energy than ever. You'll experience a fitness you can see and fitness you can feel. There's more: Creating a healthier lifestyle—and succeeding at it—has a powerfully positive effect on your self-esteem. You'll discover that your life can be fully enjoyed.

What's stopping you?

Probably reluctance to change. Most of us don't want to change. Try wearing your watch on the opposite arm and see how uncomfortable and awkward it feels. It's the same with eating new foods or starting an exercise program. It doesn't feel right, so we throw in the towel and go back to what's comfortable.

You can overcome this in three ways. First, start looking for the truth: Educate yourself about diabetes. The more you know about this disease, the better you can control it. Feeling in control helps calm the negative emotions that so often accompany any disease. What's more, if you make every effort to educate yourself about the disease, expect some rather amazing things to happen. Research shows that people who educate themselves about diabetes:

- Can get their blood sugar levels under control (which is the key to controlling diabetes)
- Can prevent the serious complications of diabetes—heart, kidney, and eye diseases
- Are highly motivated to stick to their treatment plan
- Can successfully cope with and manage the disease
- Are able to live active, quality lives with a high degree of physical and mental well-being

Clearly, you have much to gain—and nothing to lose—by simply learning as much as you can about diabetes. One way to do this is by reading the resources section at the end of this book for recommended organizations, Internet sites, publications, and books that can enhance your understanding and knowledge of diabetes.

Second, make daily, manageable resolutions, based on the advice in this book, to take better care of yourself. Your daily resolutions should be easy to pull off. Just simple, cinch stuff. Each day, when you get up, resolve two things for the day: You will eat good-for-you foods and do something active. Do this today, try it again tomorrow, and the next day, and the next. Take it day by day, but take it seriously. Before you know it, you'll be successfully controlling your diabetes and living a healthier, more vigorous life.

The third way to overcome resistance to change is to believe you can do it. If you decide there's no point in controlling your diabetes, then you're bound for trouble. Such a self-defeating attitude can pave the way to the possibility of health complications and poor quality of life.

What you think about determines what you say, what you do, and how you act. The more positive your attitude, the more successful you'll be at controlling your diabetes. There's an old saying:

What you believe, you'll achieve. Believe that you can control your diabetes, and you will.

If you're reading this book, you are probably ready to start doing just that—but you need a plan to get started. That's the goal of this book: offering step-by-step pointers that make controlling diabetes possible and easy. The six steps outlined in this book provide a workable approach that's very easy to follow, with practical suggestions to guide you at every point along the way. It's designed not only to help you control diabetes and keep it from getting worse but also to shift the disease into reverse.

In Part I, you'll learn more about diabetes—the types of diabetes, how your doctor diagnoses it, choosing the right medical team, preventing complications, the importance of regular medical care, lifesaving medical tests and medications, and the role of nutrition and exercise.

Part II describes the six steps in detail:

Step 1. Follow a Healing, Healthy Diet.

Controlling diabetes starts with a good diet. Does that mean some foods are in and some are out? Not at all. You may be pleasantly surprised to learn that there's no "diabetic diet." In fact, like most people, you get to eat a variety of foods, including your favorites. In this step, you'll learn about six simple diet principles that will help control your diabetes almost automatically.

This step also offers nutrition advice that considers your health needs, lifestyle challenges, personality, time constraints, and food preferences.

Step 2. Drive Diabetes into Retreat with Natural Remedies.

Supportive nutrients, namely, vitamins, minerals, herbs, and other natural substances, offer an appealing nondrug approach to controlling diabetes—one that can ultimately improve the quality of your life. These nutrients have remarkable healing power, which you can harness to control blood sugar, prevent diabetic complications, reduce your need for insulin, and much more. You'll be encouraged by the mounting research showing just how vital supplements are to controlling your diabetes. In this step, you'll learn which supplements work best for diabetes, how to take them, and in what amounts.

Step 3. Test Your Blood Sugar Regularly.

Checking your blood sugar level regularly is a vital step in keeping your diabetes under control. Regular testing helps ensure that your self-care program of nutrition, exercise, and medication is working. Step 3 covers what type of test to use, how to test correctly, how often to test, and how to report the results. You'll also learn about how to handle emergencies, should your blood sugar get too high or too low.

You'll need to make testing a part of your daily routine. Luckily, treating high blood sugar has never been easier. There are noninvasive (needleless) devices that accurately test your blood sugar, glucose-monitoring kits you can use in the convenience of your own home, over-the-counter products that instantly treat blood sugar problems, and other tools that will give you a take-charge attitude toward controlling your diabetes. You'll learn more about all of these.

Step 4. Get Fit to Fight Diabetes.

The more active you are, the more successful you'll be at controlling your diabetes. The combination of two forms of exercise—aerobic exercise and strength training—brings about near-miraculous effects on your body if you have diabetes. For example, both forms of exercise normalize your blood sugar, which is of primary importance in controlling diabetes. If you have to use supplemental insulin or take oral diabetes drugs, exercising may significantly reduce your requirement for insulin, depending on what type of diabetes you have, and even end the need to take oral medication. These benefits alone should be enough to get you moving!

In this step, I help you decide on the type of exercise that best suits your particular situation. Then I give you several easy-to-follow exercise routines, adaptable to your current level of fitness. When it comes to exercise, most people like to follow a set workout; they like structure. Once you have structure, there are no gray areas or room for guesswork. You know exactly what to do and how to do it. That's how the exercise routines here are set up.

Finally, I offer you some motivational tips to make exercise easy, convenient, and best of all, fun.

Step 5. Take Medicine if Your Doctor Prescribes It.

For many people, taking medicine each day is a necessity for controlling diabetes. If you have type 1 diabetes, you must take supplemental insulin to survive, because your body no longer makes insulin on its own. With type 2 diabetes, you may have to take oral diabetes pills, but usually only if diet and physical activity aren't keeping your blood sugar under control. In this step, you'll learn about diabetes medication: how it works, when to take it, and how to take it. Taking your medicine exactly as prescribed will keep your blood sugar at near-normal levels and help you live a long and active life.

Step 6. Defeat Stress with Positive Living.

Controlling your diabetes may seem like a lot to handle, bringing on stress, anxiety, and depression. But if left to linger, these emotions will get the best of you—and send your blood sugar sky-high.

Although the connection is not fully understood, the ability to handle emotions constructively, which is part of stress management, is considered an essential component of a healthy lifestyle. In this final step, you'll learn how to relieve symptoms of stress, defeat depression, conquer your fears and phobias—and get your diabetes under control as a result.

Throughout this book, you'll read about diabetes-controlling strategies contributed by leading health and medical experts who have experience in working with people like you. The advice they offer is practical, down-to-earth, and meant to improve your physical and mental health. Be sure to read it, and whenever possible, put it to practice.

So there you have it: six steps to controlling your diabetes. They can lead to a fuller, healthier, happier life. I encourage you to take these steps—and discover their life-changing, lifesaving benefits for yourself.

PART ONE

DIABETES: WHAT YOU NEED TO KNOW

Stopping a Silent Killer

If you have diabetes, take comfort in knowing that you're not alone in your challenges. In the United States, there are 16 million people with diabetes, and some 2,200 more are being diagnosed each day.

There are many more people who have diabetes but aren't even aware of it—5.4 million Americans to be exact, according to the American Diabetes Association. In fact, diabetes has been dubbed a "silent killer" because in the early stages of diabetes there are very few symptoms, or the symptoms are so mild that they don't seem to warrant serious attention. In fact, most people are unaware that they have it until diagnosed with one of its life-threatening complications, such as blindness, kidney disease, nerve disease, or cardiovascular disease. The early warning signs of diabetes are listed in the box on page 4.

Diabetes is on the rise too. Consider: While deaths from heart disease and cancer are falling, deaths from diabetes have been escalating for the past ten years. Though treatable, diabetes is the seventh leading cause of death in the United States. It contributes to nearly two hundred thousand deaths a year.

> ### EARLY WARNING SIGNS OF DIABETES
>
> Could you have diabetes and not know it? Here are the early symptoms of diabetes:
>
> - Extreme thirst
> - Unexplained hunger
> - Frequent urination
> - Unusual weight loss
> - Blurry vision
> - Unusual fatigue or drowsiness
> - Irritability
> - Tingling or numbness in the hands or feet
> - Frequent recurring skin, gum, or bladder infections
> - Slow-to-heal cuts and bruises
>
> If you notice many of these symptoms, ask your doctor if you should be tested. Early detection can delay the onset of serious diabetic complications.

Even so, there is tremendous hope. Of all life-threatening diseases, diabetes is one of easiest to get under control, because it can be managed mostly with something we all need to do: healthy living.

WHAT IS DIABETES?

For background, diabetes is a disorder of metabolism—your body's food-to-fuel process. More specifically, diabetes is a sugar metabolism disorder in which there's too much sugar (glucose) in the blood. Glucose, your body's chief fuel, is always traveling through the bloodstream. Under normal conditions, it goes from the blood into cells, where it nourishes and energizes those cells. Glucose enters the cells with the help of a hormone called insulin, which is produced by beta cells in the pancreas, a flask-shaped organ situated behind and just below the stomach.

When you eat a meal, beta cells release insulin to help your cells use and store glucose from the digestion and absorption of food. Insulin is thus the main regulator your body uses to reduce levels of glucose in the blood. Normally, blood glucose stays in the range of 70 to 115 milligrams per deciliter (mg/dl). This is the unit of measure used to describe how much glucose is in your blood at any given time.

In diabetes, though, two things can go wrong. Either the body doesn't make any or enough insulin—a condition termed *insulin deficiency*. Or cells don't respond properly to insulin—a condition called *insulin resistance*—and they receive no nourishment. In both situations, glucose is unable to enter cells, and it starts building up in the bloodstream—a condition called *hyperglycemia* or high blood sugar.

When there is too much glucose in circulation, it gums up the blood vessels that feed your organs and limbs. This is a toxic situation that provokes all sorts of metabolic problems. Blood can't travel to where it needs to go, causing problems in circulation. Your body is starved of energy, and eventually its organs deteriorate—unless blood sugar can be brought under control.

Although diabetes is often thought of as being a single disease, it is actually a family of disorders, all involving faulty metabolism of glucose. There are three major types of diabetes: type 1, type 2, and gestational diabetes.

UNDERSTANDING TYPE 1 DIABETES

Also known as insulin-dependent diabetes, type 1 diabetes is a disease in which the body either produces little insulin or no insulin at all. The disease was once called juvenile-onset diabetes, but that name has been dropped because type 1 diabetes strikes young and old alike.

Type 1 diabetes is caused by damage to the pancreas. Within the pancreas are clusters of various types of cells called islets of Langerhans. Beta cells, which make insulin, are located in the islets.

The job of the pancreas is twofold: to secrete powerful digestive enzymes for the breakdown of food and to promote the production of insulin from beta cells in the pancreas. Insulin helps glucose gain entry into cells where it is used to supply energy.

In type 1 diabetes, because the body can no longer produce insulin or make enough of it, cells cannot absorb the glucose they need for fuel. To compensate for this, the body starts breaking down proteins and digesting its own muscle tissue for fuel, resulting in muscle loss and weakness. There is also a flash flood of glucose in the blood—a surge that ultimately leads to diabetic complications. Type 1 diabetic patients, who typically get the disease at a young age, must rely on daily injections of insulin to survive.

In type 1 diabetes, insulin-producing beta cells are killed off by the body's own immune system. Upon invading the pancreas, immune cells called T cells and B cells mistake beta cells for germs and attack them—a physiological blunder referred to as an *autoimmune response*. This is why type 1 diabetes is referred to as an *autoimmune disease*. No one knows for sure why the body mounts such an attack, but researchers believe multiple forces may be at work.

RISK FACTORS FOR TYPE 1 DIABETES

Type 1 diabetes accounts for about 5 to 10 percent of those diagnosed with the disease. Major risk factors include:

- Family history. At greater risk of type 1 diabetes are children and siblings of people with the disease.

- Racial background. There is a higher incidence of type 1 diabetes among whites than is found in other racial groups.
- Age. Half of those diagnosed are under age twenty.

What causes type 1 diabetes? Here's a closer look at how type 1 diabetes may develop.

Heredity

As noted above, type 1 diabetes tends to run in families. Thus, you're at a greater risk of developing type 1 diabetes if your parents or siblings have the disease, or if you're white. Whites—particularly those of European descent—are more prone to type 1 diabetes than are people of other races.

Whether you will develop type 1 diabetes also has to do with your genes, the basic units of heredity that carry instructions for individual characteristics. Although many different types of genes may lead to the development of type 1 diabetes, researchers have pinpointed some specific genes that may predispose you to this form of the disease.

Viruses

Doctors and scientists have observed that type 1 diabetes often strikes after viral epidemics. The viruses in question include those that cause mumps and German measles. Another is the Coxsackie family of viruses, which is a close relative of the virus that causes polio.

These viruses resemble proteins found in the beta cells of the pancreas. In a bodily sort of "friendly fire," the immune system mistakes beta cells for virus particles and obliterates them, along with their ability to manufacture insulin.

Cow's Milk

Some researchers suspect that exposure to cow's milk during infancy may trigger an autoimmune response leading to type 1 diabetes. This theory cropped up after studies revealed that children newly diagnosed with type 1 diabetes often had high levels of antibodies to a specific protein found in cow's milk. This protein is called bovine serum albumin (BSA), and it resembles a protein found in beta cells.

The intestines of babies in the first several months of life cannot properly break down or digest certain foods, including proteins. These large, undigested proteins pass through the intestines into the bloodstream. The body considers such proteins, including BSA, as foreign invaders and creates antibodies to attack them. In a case of a biochemical mistaken identity, those same antibodies attack beta cells because they look like BSA.

To date, research has found that infants fed cow's milk during their first three months of life are one and a half times more likely to develop type 1 diabetes. However, some research shows no link between cow's milk and the development of the disease. In response to such contradictory findings, scientists emphasize that more studies are needed to verify a connection and to firmly establish whether there is a true risk associated with feeding cow's milk to infants.

Free Radicals

Some diabetes investigators theorize that free-radical damage may contribute to type 1 diabetes. Free radicals are unstable molecules generated by metabolism, respiration, stress, environmental pollutants, and other factors. They injure cell membranes, making it easy for bacteria, viruses, and other disease-causing agents to slip in and inflict harm. Free radicals can destroy cells, tissues, and even organs, weakening the immune system and leaving the body vulnerable to a range of diseases.

Normally, your body has a built-in brigade of natural substances, including enzymes, that prevent free-radical damage. But in type 1 diabetes, cells in the pancreas are naturally low in levels of these protective enzymes. Unchecked, free radicals can run rampant and decimate beta cells.

Fortunately, though, powerful nutrients called antioxidants, found in foods and nutritional supplements, can snuff out free radicals, fortify internal enzyme defenses, and protect the body against needless damage. For more information on antioxidants, see Step 2.

Chemicals and Drugs

Research indicates that exposure to or ingestion of certain chemicals and drugs can trigger type 1 diabetes. One of these is Pyriminil, a rat poison. Others are pentamidine, used to treat pneumonia; and L-asparaginase, an anticancer agent. Other chemicals have been shown to cause diabetes in animals, but researchers aren't yet sure whether they do the same in people.

Because diabetes is so complex, it is unlikely that a single drug or chemical causes the disease by itself. Rather, exposure to drugs or chemicals may activate diabetes if you are already genetically susceptible to the disease.

MAJOR TREATMENTS

The cornerstone for treating type 1 diabetes is insulin, which is available in several different strengths and forms. Insulin replaces the insulin your body can no longer produce. Your physician will specify which kind of insulin to take, how much, and when. Information on how to use insulin is provided in Step 4.

Insulin alone won't control your diabetes. Other approaches are necessary too. These include:

- Meal planning that focuses on low-fat nutrition, moderate amounts of protein, and designated quantities of high-fiber, complex carbohydrates. Your diet must also be consistent; that is, you must eat roughly the same amount of calories each day, eat meals and snacks at the same time every day, and not miss meals.
- Exercise that includes both strength training and aerobics to help your cells take in glucose, to build muscle, and to prevent diabetic complications.
- Regular blood sugar checks to keep track of how you're doing.
- Stress management to ensure that your body's own immunity and healing power are not hampered by stress and other health-defeating emotions.

Once you start following these strategies on a day-to-day basis, controlling your diabetes will become second nature. The new habits you adopt will improve many other aspects of your health, and you'll be a healthier person for it.

UNDERSTANDING TYPE 2 DIABETES

Also called non-insulin-dependent diabetes, type 2 diabetes is the most common form of the disease, accounting for 90 to 95 percent of all cases. You may have heard that this type of diabetes is not so serious as type 1. That is a myth. Both types of diabetes put you at a higher-than-average risk for heart attack, stroke, kidney disease, and other serious complications.

There are some important differences between type 2 and type 1 diabetes, however. In type 1 diabetes, your body is unable to produce insulin, or there isn't enough insulin to go around. In type 2 diabetes, the body makes insulin, but the cells have trouble using it.

For insulin to work, it has to access cells by first attaching to special proteins on cell membranes called *receptors*, which have two important functions with regard to glucose. First, receptors operate like door locks. Once insulin gets to the receptor, it acts like a key and unlocks the receptors surrounding the cell. The cell opens up and lets glucose in for use as fuel. Second, insulin receptors signal another type of protein, called a glucose transporter, to carry glucose into the cell.

In type 2 diabetes, things go awry with the entire entrance process. In some cases, the "locks" don't work, and cells ignore—or become resistant to—the insulin. This condition is termed *insulin resistance*. Because of insulin resistance, insulin can't open the cell. Glucose is locked out, and it clutters up the bloodstream. The pancreas is forced to pump out more insulin to handle the excess glucose in the blood. But eventually, the pancreas can't keep pace with the demand. These events ultimately lead to risky complications.

In other cases, there are too few insulin receptors on cells, or insulin simply doesn't perform the job it is supposed to do. Whatever the problem, glucose can't get into the cell. Also, in some people with type 2 diabetes, beta cells do not manufacture enough insulin.

RISK FACTORS FOR TYPE 2 DIABETES

Risk factors for type 2 diabetes are linked largely to age, diet, and lifestyle, although genetic factors are involved too. Specific risk factors include:

- Obesity.
- A sedentary lifestyle.
- A diagnosis of impaired glucose tolerance (IGT) as a result of a fasting plasma glucose test and an oral glucose tolerance test. IGT is a condition in which your glucose levels are abnormally elevated but are not high enough to indicate full-blown diabetes.
- Syndrome X, an abnormal metabolic condition.
- Abnormal levels of blood fats in your system.
- Ethnic heritage (African Americans, Latinos, Asian and Pacific Islanders, and American Indians are at greater risk).
- Having had *gestational diabetes*, a rare form of diabetes that develops during pregnancy but disappears afterward.
- Having given birth to a baby weighing nine pounds or more.

What follows is a closer look at some of the key factors involved in the development of type 2 diabetes.

Heredity

Your chance of type 2 diabetes catching up with you down the road may depend on your genes. Like type 1 diabetes, type 2 diabetes runs in families. In fact, there may be an even stronger genetic component involved in type 2 diabetes than in type 1 diabetes, an observation that has been substantiated in studies of twins. Researchers have found that if an identical twin develops type 1 diabetes, there is a 25 to 50 percent chance that the other twin will get the disease too. On the other hand, if an identical twin develops type 2 diabetes, there is a 60 to 75 percent chance that the other twin will develop it as well.

Evidence for a genetic component has been observed in studies of ethnic groups. Compared to whites, type 2 diabetes occurs more often in African Americans, Hispanics (with the exception of Cuban Americans), Asian Americans, Pacific Islanders, and American Indians. In fact, American Indians have the highest rates of diabetes in the world.

While it is clear that genes play a significant role in the development of type 2 diabetes, no specific genes have yet been identified. Researchers, however, are finding "errors" in genes that make body cells unresponsive to insulin. They also suspect the existence of an obesity gene, meaning that some people may be genetically inclined to obesity. Obesity is the number-one cause of type 2 diabetes.

Obesity

One reason diabetes may be on the rise is the escalating rate of obesity in the United States, which has one of the highest rates of obesity in the world. According to a national survey, nearly 74 percent of Americans age twenty-five or older are overweight.

Your odds of developing type 2 diabetes climb as your weight climbs. Weighing at least 20 percent more than what is recommended for your height and build puts you in the *obese* category. More than 80 percent of people with type 2 diabetes are obese. For reasons that have not yet been fully spelled out by research, excess pudge causes insulin resistance. Body cells, in effect, ignore insulin, and the hormone cannot ease glucose into cells.

Where you carry your weight makes a difference too. If you have an apple shape, or "central obesity," which is characterized by excess abdominal fat, you're at a greater risk of developing type 2 diabetes than those with fat deposited mostly on their hips ("pear shape").

Here's the reason: Fat storage areas near the abdominal muscles liberate a lot of excess fat into the bloodstream in the form of fatty acids. This surplus of fatty acids in circulation wreaks all sorts of havoc. Muscle cells become less sensitive to insulin; the liver can't break down insulin properly, and so it begins making more glucose. Collectively, this situation causes insulin, glucose, and fat levels to rise—all factors that can aggravate type 2 diabetes or hasten its development.

The strong connection between type 2 diabetes and obesity is the main reason why nutrition and exercise are the primary treatments for this form of the disease. Thus, weight loss through diet and regular exercise is essential to getting rid of health-ruining fat and controlling type 2 diabetes.

Inactivity

In the United States today, about 27 percent of us are considered sedentary—in other words, we're couch potatoes—and 33 percent of us are on-again off-again exercisers. Very few people get enough exercise to improve their health and well-being. Small wonder, then, that so many chronic illnesses—including diabetes—are on a deadly ascent in our society.

Leading an inactive lifestyle contributes to type 2 diabetes and expedites its progression in two likely ways. First, inactivity leads to obesity, which is the major promoter of type 2 diabetes. Second, inactivity makes body cells resistant to using insulin and taking in glucose.

By contrast, exercise encourages insulin use by stimulating a protein inside muscle cells that carries glucose into these cells.

Because muscle cells are the hungriest consumers of glucose, they must also rely heavily on insulin. Thus, priming insulin action is a vital function of exercise. In Step 4, you'll learn more about how to use exercise to control glucose levels.

Syndrome X

This rather mysterious-sounding condition sets the stage for both type 2 diabetes and cardiovascular disease. It is characterized by a cluster of symptoms:

- Glucose intolerance, which occurs when insulin can't effectively usher glucose into cells.
- Central obesity. As explained, abdominal fat releases a lot of fatty acids into circulation where they initiate all sorts of mischief. These fatty acids make muscle cells less sensitive to insulin as well as disturb the liver's ability to break down insulin. As a result, the liver begins churning out too much glucose, along with artery-clogging lipids.
- Hyperlipidemia, a combination of elevated triglycerides and reduced HDL cholesterol in the blood.
- High blood pressure.

How does Syndrome X develop? Diet is mostly to blame, particularly one that's high in refined carbohydrates such as sweets, breads, and processed snack foods. Such foods trigger a rapid spike in blood sugar, and the body responds by pumping more insulin into the bloodstream to handle the sugar. Over time, insulin levels in your blood remain higher than they should be. This promotes fat storage, elevates blood fats, and raises blood pressure.

The upshot of these metabolic problems is type 2 diabetes and heart disease. Happily, though, Syndrome X can be prevented and reversed with weight loss, regular exercise, low-fat foods, and a switch from refined foods to natural choices such as fruits, vegetables, and whole grains.

Age

With advancing age, your body gradually loses its ability to regulate glucose. At the same time, many people become less physically active as they get older and gain weight as a result. These situations put you in danger of developing type 2 diabetes, which typically occurs in people over forty-five years old, particularly among those who are overweight. Nearly 11 percent of Americans age sixty-five to seventy-four have type 2 diabetes. What's more, the disease is present in 25 percent of the population age eighty-five and older.

On the surface, it may look like type 2 diabetes is a middle-age or geriatric disease. Alarmingly, though, type 2 diabetes is on the rise among children and teenagers. Some recent data indicate that since the 1980s, there has been a 54 percent increase in the prevalence of type 2 diabetes among teenagers and a 45 percent increase among children. The reason for such a steep rise is the growing rate of obesity among our nation's youth.

Free Radicals

With type 2 diabetes, you may have low levels of internally produced antioxidants in your body. Antioxidants are a group of beneficial substances that squelch free radicals and prevent them from inflicting bodily harm. When antioxidants are in short supply, free radicals take over and attack tissues. This may contribute to type 2 diabetes and ultimately lead to complications.

Smoking

Each year, smoking kills approximately four hundred thousand Americans—primarily due to lung cancer, chronic lung disease, and heart attack. Now researchers have discovered a strong link between chronic cigarette smoking and type 2 diabetes. Although smoking doesn't directly cause type 2 diabetes, it intensifies insulin resistance in chronic smokers. So if you're a smoker suffering from type 2 diabetes, you're adding insult to injury by continuing to light up. Smoking inflicts further damage on your body's already poor insulin response.

The chief culprit in insulin resistance appears to be nicotine, the drug in tobacco. This was discovered in studies of people using nicotine patches and gum to kick the habit. Researchers found that these forms of nicotine, like cigarettes, made body cells less responsive to insulin. Smoking also generates free radicals, which can do irreparable harm to your body.

MAJOR TREATMENTS

Controlling type 2 diabetes involves a lifestyle fix in which your goal is to lower glucose and improve your body's use of insulin. The wonderful news is that you can accomplish this mostly with diet, exercise, and other nondrug measures. For example:

- Meal planning that focuses on low-fat nutrition, moderate amounts of protein, and designated quantities of high-fiber, complex carbohydrates
- Weight loss to help your body use insulin better and bring your diabetes under control
- Regular blood sugar checks to keep track of how you're doing

- Exercise that includes both resistance training and aerobics to stimulate normal insulin activity helps your cells take in glucose, assists you in burning body fat, and prevents diabetic complications

In some cases, healthy habits such as good nutrition, exercise, and weight control are not enough. Your physician may prescribe oral diabetes medications or insulin shots. Not everyone with type 2 diabetes takes pills or insulin, however.

All of the major ways to control type 1 and type 2 diabetes are covered in detail in the six steps outlined later in this book. The key point to remember is that controlling diabetes is not a program but a long-term way of living.

UNDERSTANDING GESTATIONAL DIABETES

A less common form of diabetes is gestational diabetes, which develops only in pregnant women with no previous history of diabetes. Approximately 135,000 women in the United States develop gestational diabetes each year.

Gestational diabetes is most likely caused by hormones from the placenta that are involved in baby's growth. These hormones may block the mother's ability to properly use insulin, leading to insulin resistance.

In addition, some women are genetically susceptible to gestational diabetes. Researchers speculate that the gene for gestational diabetes and type 2 diabetes may be similar.

Gestational diabetes develops when your body is unable to produce and use all the insulin it requires for pregnancy—which is up to three times as much insulin as when you're not pregnant. As with other forms of diabetes, glucose builds up in your bloodstream.

Untreated or poorly controlled gestational diabetes can cause problems for you and your developing baby. The excess glucose in your bloodstream passes through the placenta into your baby's system. Consequently, your baby's pancreas starts churning out extra insulin to dispose of the glucose. This can cause a condition termed *macrosomia*, or "fat" baby. Giving birth to a very large baby may necessitate a cesarean section delivery. Macrosomia puts your child at risk of low blood sugar at birth, a major cause of breathing problems. Also, babies with too much insulin are at risk for obesity as children. Further, the odds are greater that they will develop type 2 diabetes as adults.

If pregnant, you should be screened for gestational diabetes between your twenty-fourth and twenty-eighth week of pregnancy, particularly if you have the following risk factors:

- You are twenty-five years old or older.
- You were overweight before becoming pregnant.
- You have a family history of diabetes.
- You are Hispanic, African American, American Indian, Asian American, or a Pacific Islander.

To test for gestational diabetes, your physician will measure your blood sugar response to glucose ingested in a drink. If you have gestational diabetes, your physician may prescribe daily blood sugar testing and insulin injections. Normally, though, gestational diabetes clears up on its own.

If it goes away by itself, then why should you care about it? Gestational diabetes may return in future pregnancies. In addition, research indicates that about 40 percent of women with gestational diabetes develop type 2 diabetes within about fifteen years.

Fortunately, gestational diabetes and type 2 diabetes are preventable in many cases and manageable in cases where there may be a genetic link. Watching your weight during pregnancy, eating healthy foods, and following a sensible program of exercise will help minimize insulin resistance and prevent gestational diabetes. If you take these measures, you should have a healthy pregnancy, a healthy start for your new baby, and a healthy life in general.

HOW TO BEAT THE ODDS

A research survey asked people with diabetes: "What has been most difficult about living with diabetes?" Seventy-four percent responded "controlling the disease."

If you feel the same way, take heart: Diabetes may not be curable, but it is manageable. Through proper diet, supplementation, exercise, consistent self-care, and emotional fitness, you can successfully control your diabetes. What's more, the sooner you start controlling your diabetes and preventing its complications, the greater your chance of keeping the disease in check—and living a full, vigorous, and healthy life.

• • •

WHAT THE EXPERTS ADVISE
Top-Ten Strategies for Learning About Your Diabetes

Sherrye Landrum, associate director, Consumer Books
American Diabetes Association

The American Diabetes Association is the nation's leading voluntary health organization supporting diabetes research, information, and advocacy. Its mission is to prevent and cure diabetes and to improve the lives of all people affected by diabetes. Here are the association's tips for learning about diabetes.

1. Ask your doctor, diabetes educator, and dietitian more questions than you've ever asked before in your life. This disease is yours. The way it is managed is up to you. The details of lifestyle, food likes and dislikes, daily schedule, exercise, and family and cultural expectations will color how you and diabetes interact. No one else has diabetes like you have it. You're the expert on you. Now you need to become an expert in diabetes too.

2. Write a list of questions for your doctor or endocrinologist. Keep a running list. When you only have about fifteen minutes with your health care provider, you may forget what you meant to ask.

3. Go to the library and read everything it has about diabetes, healthy eating, and exercise written in the past five years. Books provide both education and motivation. The more you know, the healthier you'll be—today and in the future.

4. Put your knowledge into action. Getting your blood sugar nearer to normal can prevent or delay most of the complications of diabetes. It's worth the investment in time and energy to learn how to do it. And because you keep growing and changing, the information you need will change, too.

5. Join organizations such as the American Diabetes Association (ADA) that support diabetes research and provide you with the latest information about new treatment choices. They are working to find a cure! They will provide you with free information to help you get started dealing with your diabetes as soon as you call or E-mail them.

6. Subscribe to magazines such as *Diabetes Forecast* to keep up to date about the latest developments in diabetes care and research. Monthly columns and articles help you tackle the everyday details of meal planning and exercise that keep you healthier and help you stay motivated. You will be amazed at the wide world of people and events that diabetes touches.

7. There are lots of Web sites offering information about diabetes. Aim for quality sites from respected organizations in the field, such as the ADA, the Joslin Diabetes Centers, the National Institute of Diabetes and Digestive and Kidney Diseases at the National Institutes of Health, and the Centers for Disease Control and Prevention.

8. Enroll in a local diabetes education class. Several years later, enroll in another one. Several years later, enroll in another. It's vital to your health to return for a knowledge tune-up and to hear the latest news. For example, did you know that people with diabetes can eat sugar? Being diagnosed with diabetes is a shock. You cannot absorb all you need to know about living well with this disease in the first year of it. Use every means possible to learn something new about diabetes at least once a month.

9. Whenever you have a life change, such as going off to college, getting a new job, getting pregnant, a vacation to a faraway place, or retirement, you need to learn how to smoothly fit your diabetes into it. A certified diabetes educator is your best friend in these situations—and can help you design a new meal plan too. A CDE has passed a national exam in diabetes education and is knowledgeable in diabetes care.

10. Use the information that you gather about your diabetes to learn more about yourself. The results of your daily blood glucose checks and your regular glycohemoglobin tests help you make decisions about your food choices, exercise, and diabetes medication.

Unmasking Trouble: How Your Doctor Diagnoses Diabetes

Whether you actually have diabetes can be confirmed only by your doctor after conducting a thorough physical examination and running specific tests that determine the levels of glucose in your blood. It's helpful to understand how your doctor diagnoses diabetes, so that you can feel confident about the process and be able to ask questions about it. Remember: The more you know about your diabetes—including tests and test results—the better you can keep it under control. To help you, here's a rundown of the major tests used to diagnose diabetes.

BLOOD TESTS

Used to diagnose all major forms of diabetes, blood tests determine whether you have too-high levels of glucose in your blood. There are two general types of blood tests: *screening tests* and *diagnostic tests*.

Screening tests, which are performed on people with no symptoms of diabetes, take a drop of blood from your fingertip. The blood is analyzed on the spot, and the results are ready within minutes. Available in doctors' offices or at health fairs, a screening test should be given if you have risk factors for diabetes.

Your doctor will perform a diagnostic test if diabetes is suspected, based on your symptoms or on the results of a screening test. A blood sample is collected from your vein and sent to a laboratory for analysis. There are three types of diagnostic tests used to confirm a diagnosis of diabetes:

Fasting plasma glucose test. Among the three diagnostic tests, this blood test is the preferred way to test for diabetes and is considered the standard. After you have fasted overnight for at least eight hours, a sample of your blood is drawn at your doctor's office and sent to a lab for analysis.

After fasting, normal plasma glucose levels are less than 100 milligrams per deciliter (mg/dl). But if fasting plasma glucose levels exceed 126 mg/dl, your doctor will suspect diabetes. A firmer diagnosis can be made when two fasting plasma glucose tests, performed on different days, are above 126 mg/dl. According to the American Diabetes Association, you can be diagnosed with diabetes if your glucose is at least 126 mg/dl on two or more occasions.

Random plasma glucose test. This is the simplest way to detect diabetes. The test measures glucose in your blood at any given time and is conducted without fasting. It is used to test for diabetes when symptoms exist. Blood samples showing a blood glucose level of 200 mg/dl or higher are a sign of diabetes. The results of a random plasma glucose test, however, must be reconfirmed at another time with a fasting plasma glucose or an oral glucose tolerance test.

Oral glucose tolerance test. With this test, you go without food for at least eight but not more than sixteen hours. The next morning at the doctor's office or laboratory, your fasting plasma glucose is tested. After that test, you ingest a measured amount of liquid glucose.

Your blood glucose levels are then measured five times over a period of three hours to see how fast they rise and fall. In people without diabetes, glucose levels rise, then fall quickly. If you have diabetes, glucose levels rise more rapidly than normal but do not fall as fast.

To check glucose levels, a lab technician or nurse collects blood from a vein in your arm. Blood is drawn every hour until your blood glucose level returns to normal. The test takes approximately two to three hours.

For the oral glucose tolerance test to be reliable, you must be in relatively good health and be normally active. The morning of the test, you should not be on any drugs (including caffeine and nicotine) that could affect the test. For three days prior to the test, you should eat a diet high in carbohydrates (about 150 to 200 grams a day).

A normal response to an oral glucose tolerance test is a measurement of less than 140 mg/dl at the two-hour mark, and measurements of less than 200 mg/dl between zero and two hours.

A suspicious number is a sustained value of greater than or equal to 200 mg/dl. This usually indicates diabetes.

You may be diagnosed with impaired glucose tolerance (IGT) if your fasting plasma glucose is less than 126 mg/dl and your two-hour glucose level is between 140 and 199 mg/dl. IGT is a condition in which glucose levels are higher than normal but not high enough to be classified as diabetes. IGT is present in about 11 percent of adults, roughly 20 million Americans. It is a specific risk factor for type 2 diabetes. You can prevent IGT with many of the same lifestyle recommendations discussed in this book.

If you are pregnant, your doctor may test you for gestational diabetes, a pregnancy-related form of the disease. You will be diagnosed with gestational diabetes if you have any two of the following:

- A fasting plasma glucose level of more than 95 mg/dl
- A one-hour glucose level of more than 180 mg/dl
- A two-hour glucose level of more than 155 mg/dl
- A three-hour glucose level of more than 140 mg/dl

Your doctor will explain what the results of your blood tests mean. Again, be sure to ask questions if you do not understand the results. You have the right and responsibility to ask for clarification. It's your health that's at stake.

Preventing Life-Threatening Complications

If diabetes goes undiagnosed or is allowed to rage out of control long enough, serious—even deadly—complications can arise. But by keeping your diabetes under control, you can put a powerful roadblock in the path of these complications.

So that you understand the health consequences of poorly controlled diabetes, here is a closer look at the major complications of the disease and how to prevent them.

COMPLICATIONS OF DIABETES

Heart Disease

Heart disease is the leading cause of death in people who suffer from diabetes. In fact, the death toll among diabetics with heart disease is about two to four times higher than in adults without diabetes. The reason is that people with diabetes often have high levels of lipids (cholesterol and triglycerides) and thus are at greater risk of developing atherosclerosis, the narrowing and thickening of the arteries. What's more, excess glucose in the blood accelerates atherosclerosis. Blood flow to the heart slows down or is shut off altogether.

A symptom of reduced blood flow to the heart is angina, or chest pain. It is often the first warning sign of coronary heart disease. A heart attack occurs when blood flow to the heart is completely cut off, and part of the heart muscle dies.

In poorly controlled diabetes, reduced blood flow can affect other parts of the body too. In the legs and feet, for example, poor circulation leads to *intermittent claudification*, characterized by leg pain and leg cramps. If circulation problems persist and worsen in the legs and feet, the result can be chronic ulcers, numbness, and in severe cases, gangrene, which can necessitate amputation of the affected limb.

Stroke

Stroke is the lightning bolt of circulatory diseases—striking without much warning. It is a disturbance to the brain's blood supply, caused by a blood clot or by a ruptured blood vessel that bleeds into the brain. The risk of stroke is two to four times higher in diabetics.

Stroke in diabetes is caused by the same mechanism that damages coronary arteries: too much fat and glucose in the blood. Blood vessels narrow and become plugged, and the blood supply to the brain is disrupted. Starved, brain cells either die or stop functioning. When that happens, the jobs they do—vision, movement, and speech—cease or are impaired.

High Blood Pressure

Nearly 60 to 65 percent of people with diabetes have high blood pressure (hypertension), meaning a blood pressure reading above 140/90. However, medical experts don't know which comes first:

diabetes or hypertension. Nor do they know exactly why diabetes keeps such close company with hypertension. But there are some theories. Factors that may give rise to high blood pressure in diabetes may include insulin resistance (in type 2 diabetes), obesity, and excess secretion of stress hormones.

Another factor has to do with sodium (salt), which can raise blood pressure. The salt–blood pressure connection can be more dangerous in people with diabetes than in those without the disease. That's because many people with diabetes tend to be *sodium sensitive*, which means they can get a rise in blood pressure at low daily salt intakes. Cutting back on salt is a good idea for everyone; it is especially recommended if you have diabetes.

With high blood pressure, blood shoots through the arteries at a dangerous pressure, like water gushing through pipes at full tilt. The heart is thus forced to work overtime, a situation that damages the interior lining of the arteries. Untreated, high blood pressure may eventually lead to the development of a fatty tissue called *arthernoma* inside arteries. This can constrict or obstruct the arteries. High blood pressure also damages tiny blood vessels feeding your eyes, kidneys, and other organs.

Retinopathy and Other Eye Diseases

Diabetes can usher in a condition called diabetic retinopathy, a disease of the retina, which is a thin membrane attached to the back of your eye. Like the film in a camera, the retina senses and processes light images projected through your eyes.

Usually occurring in both eyes, diabetic retinopathy is caused by the progressive deterioration of blood vessels that supply blood to the retina. Diabetes weakens the walls of these blood vessels, and sometimes the vessels break, causing hemorrhages within the retina or other parts of the eye. The hemorrhages cloud vision. The

CATEGORIES OF BLOOD PRESSURE FOR ADULTS AGE 18 AND OLDER

CATEGORY	SYSTOLIC	DIASTOLIC
Normal	130 or below	85 or below
High normal	130–139	85–89

High blood pressure:
  Stage 1 (mild)
  Stage 2 (moderate)
  Stage 3 (severe)
  Stage 4 (very severe)
	
	140–159
	160–179
	180–209
	Above 210
		
		90–99
		100–109
		110–119
		Above 120

Blood pressure is categorized according to stages of severity, as the chart shows. The only way to detect high blood pressure is to have it taken regularly. With each contraction of the heart, the pressure of the blood in the arteries reaches a peak, called the systolic pressure. Then the pressure gradually decreases to a minimum, the diastolic pressure, before the next contraction. Blood pressure is always expressed as two numbers. Normal blood pressure, for example, is 130/85 or below. The top number is the systolic pressure; the bottom number is the diastolic pressure.

Both numbers are important. Many people believe that a high systolic pressure is harmless when the diastolic pressure is low. But recent research indicates that high systolic pressure leads to the same complications of high blood pressure, namely stroke and heart attack.

Source: Stenger, A. 1993. New guidelines for hypertension. *The Physician and Sportsmedicine,* 21: 55–56.

retina often absorbs the blood, a process that leads to scarring. The scars decrease vision. This type of retinopathy is termed *nonproliferative* (or background) retinopathy. It usually does not cause blindness unless blood leaks into the macula, an area of the retina near the optic nerve.

A less common form of retinopathy is *proliferative* retinopathy. This occurs when new blood vessels grow over the retina and into the vitreous humor, the jellylike substance in the back of the eye. These blood vessels are abnormal and can sprout uncontrollably.

Further, they rupture easily, causing loss of vision. Proliferative retinopathy promotes the formation of scar tissue on the retina. This scar tissue can shrivel, causing the layers of the retina to tear apart.

Retinopathy can also cause the macula of the eye to swell—a condition termed *macular edema*. The macula, which is located in the middle of the retina, lets you see fine detail. Macular swelling leads to impaired vision and blindness.

Retinopathy is usually diagnosed in people who have had diabetes for at least ten years. Nearly all people with diabetes show symptoms of retinopathy after thirty years of living with the disease. On average, twelve thousand to twenty-four thousand new cases of diabetic retinopathy are diagnosed annually.

Diabetes can also lead to glaucoma, or high blood pressure within the eye. Cataracts, in which the normally clear lens of the eye becomes clouded, are also more common in people with diabetes.

Nephropathy (Kidney Disease)

Diabetic nephropathy is a deterioration of the small blood vessels, and sometimes the nerves, in the kidneys, a pair of bean-shaped organs located against the back of the abdominal wall. It is the job of the kidneys to filter out toxins that the body makes or takes in. Tiny filtering units called nephrons perform this task.

Too much glucose in the blood places a strain on the nephrons and thickens their membranes, jeopardizing their ability to filter out toxins. Blood vessels associated with the nephrons leak and become blocked. Some of the toxins that should be filtered out remain in your blood, while important substances such as protein and nutrients are lost in urine instead of staying put in the blood. If your doctor finds an excess of protein in your urine during a routine physical, diabetes may be suspected.

When blood glucose levels reach 200 mg/dl, your kidneys can

no longer reabsorb sugar. Consequently, it spills out into your urine. Sugar attracts water. So when sugar is excreted from the body, it pulls water along with it. This causes the frequent urination, excessive thirst, and weight loss that are signs of diabetes.

Not everyone with diabetes gets nephropathy, although about a third do. If diabetic-related kidney disease is advanced, a condition known as *end-stage renal disease* results. This means that the kidneys are failing and can no longer filter out impurities. End-stage renal disease is treated by either kidney dialysis, in which a machine does the job kidneys are supposed to do; or kidney transplantation, in which the patient receives a new kidney.

Neuropathy (Nervous System Disease)

Although it is not clear why, diabetes damages nerve cells, or neurons, the basic units of the nervous system that are responsible for the transmission of messages at great speed. Scientists believe that excess glucose in the blood may disturb the chemical balance inside nerves, or that the blood supply to nerves may be shut off and nerve cells become starved for oxygen.

Whatever the reason, damaged nerves lead to a host of problems, including pain in the extremities or other parts of the body, impaired sensation in the limbs, tingling, numbness, poor digestion, loss of bladder or bowel control, and impotence.

There are three types of neuropathy:

- Distal symmetric neuropathy affects nerves in your arms, hands, feet, or legs on both sides of your body. Symptoms include numbness, loss of sensitivity to heat and cold, muscular weakness, tingling, or pain.
- Focal neuropathy is a rare form of neuropathy resulting from damage to a single nerve or a group of nerves. It devel-

ops when blood flow to a nerve is choked off due to the obstruction of a vessel feeding that particular nerve. Symptoms include pain, loss of feeling, and poor muscular coordination in the affected area.

- Autonomic neuropathy can affect countless bodily functions. Involuntary actions such as heartbeat, respiration, and digestion are regulated by a part of the nervous system called the autonomic nervous system. When nerves in this system are damaged, the result is autonomic neuropathy. Stomach muscles, for example, can slow down or become inefficient, resulting in diarrhea or vomiting. Damage to nerves involved in bladder function can lead to poor bladder control or inability to empty the bladder. If urine stays in your bladder too long, you run the risk of urinary tract infections. Impotence is a result of autonomic neuropathy too.

About 60 to 70 percent of diabetics have mild to severe forms of damage to the nervous system. Sadly, severe forms of diabetic nerve damage can necessitate the need for lower limb amputation.

Infections

With diabetes, you are particularly susceptible to infections, for several reasons. To begin with, excess glucose in the blood jeopardizes the job of your immune cells, which normally attack invading bacteria, viruses, and fungi that cause infections. Even worse, these invading organisms love to snack on the extra glucose in your blood, increasing the spread of infection. To make matters worse, infections are likely to heal more slowly than normal because of impaired circulation.

In diabetes, the areas of the body most prone to infection are the mouth and gums, skin, legs and feet, urinary tract, vagina, and respiratory tract.

PREVENTING AND TREATING COMPLICATIONS

Some encouraging news: About 20 to 30 percent of people with diabetes never get serious complications. But since the risk of complications exists, the best way to reduce it is to keep your blood sugar under control. That's because most of the complications of diabetes are caused by excess glucose in the blood. Controlling blood sugar—which ultimately controls your diabetes—is the focus of the steps in this book. But it is vital to add here that there are other measures you can take to prevent and treat complications, and these are summarized in the box on page 36.

PREVENTION AND TREATMENT OF DIABETIC COMPLICATIONS

COMPLICATION	PREVENTION	TREATMENT
Heart disease	• Control glucose • Stop smoking • Follow a low-fat diet • Control body weight • Control blood pressure • Exercise	• Surgery to remove blockages • Medication • Dietary therapy • Exercise
Stroke	• Control glucose • Stop smoking • Follow a low-fat diet • Control body weight • Control blood pressure • Exercise	• Surgery • Rehabilitation • Medication • Dietary therapy • Exercise
High blood pressure	• Control glucose • Stop smoking • Follow a low-fat diet • Control body weight • Control blood pressure • Exercise	• Medication • Dietary therapy • Exercise
Retinopathy and other eye diseases	• Control glucose • Have yearly eye exams	• Laser treatment called *photocoagulation* that destroys abnormal blood vessels and slows the formation of new ones • Eye drops (for glaucoma) • Surgery (for glaucoma) • Surgery (for cataracts)
Nephropathy	• Control glucose • Control blood pressure by maintaining a healthy weight and avoiding too much salt	• Blood pressure medication • Low-protein diet • Kidney dialysis • Kidney transplant

PREVENTION AND TREATMENT OF DIABETIC COMPLICATIONS (cont'd)		
COMPLICATION	**PREVENTION**	**TREATMENT**
Nervous system disease	• Control glucose • Control blood pressure • Stop smoking • Follow a healthy diet • Minimize alcohol intake • Exercise	• Medication • Topical ointments to ease pain • Special footwear
Infection	• Control glucose • Regular brushing and flossing (to prevent gum disease) • Wear cotton underwear (to prevent vaginal infections) • Conduct regular self-examinations for foot problems • Exercise to promote blood flow to feet • Stop smoking (to improve blood flow to feet) • Control blood pressure and high cholesterol (to improve blood flow to feet)	• Dental surgery (for advanced gum disease) • Antifungal cream (for vaginal infections) • Amputation (for out-of-control foot and leg infection)

Choosing Quality Caregivers

Controlling your diabetes and preventing its complications result primarily from the day-to-day activities you do to stay healthy, from nutritious eating to regular exercise. But there's also medical care to consider. Although you're in charge of the daily management of your diabetes, you need to be under the care of a great doctor—someone with competency, compassion, and communication skills.

How do you find such a doctor?

One way is to compile a thorough checklist. So let's get started.

Specialist. To begin with, you'll want to be treated by a physician who specializes in diabetes. That physician is responsible for the medical management of your diabetes, including insulin or oral diabetes drugs, and the detection and treatment of complications.

Recommendations. Get a recommendation from your primary care physician (if he or she will not be treating your diabetes) for a physician who specializes in diabetes (a diabetologist) or for an endocrinologist, a physician who also treats diabetes and other metabolic diseases.

In addition, talk to other people with diabetes to find out which doctors they recommend. Ask medical professionals such as hospital nurses, pharmacists, dentists, and others. They are a good source of insider information on physicians. Finally, contact diabetes support groups in your community or chapters of your local American Diabetes Association for recommendations.

Special training or recognition in diabetes care. Ideally, locate a physician who is in the American Diabetes Association Provider Recognition Program, made up of approximately twelve hundred primary care physicians and diabetes specialists who have received recognition for setting high standards and performance levels in diabetes care. These physicians have proved that they do an exceptional job of caring for patients with diabetes and assessing diabetic complications. You can get in touch with the Provider Recognition Program by calling (703) 549-1500, ext. 2202, or logging on to www.diabetes.org/recognition.

Board certificate. Check the doctor's credentials to be sure that he or she is board-certified, since board certification indicates that physicians are exceptionally qualified in their fields of medicine and stay current in their specialties. If you are looking for a specialist, you want a doctor who is board-certified in endocrinology or internal medicine.

Hospital affiliations. Check out the hospitals in your area. Good doctors are usually affiliated with good hospitals. You can find out this information by calling the doctor's office, then verifying it with the hospital.

First impressions. Schedule a get-acquainted appointment. It will give you enough facts and firsthand information to help you decide if you want to become this doctor's patient. (As with any doctor visit, you'll pay a fee.) Observe the following:

- Is the office staff courteous and efficient when you call to make your appointment? The way you're treated by the staff

can be an indicator of how the doctor will treat you, since the moods of the front-office people are often shaped by their boss.
- Once you get there, do you have to wait a long time before seeing the doctor? A wait of more than fifteen minutes *without an explanation* is unreasonable. There may, however, be a good reason. A doctor who takes extra time with one patient probably will give you extra time when necessary.
- Is the doctor friendly and responsive, or preoccupied? A good physician can comfort and communicate with his or her patients. If these qualities aren't there, shop around for another doctor.
- Find out the doctor's approach to treating diabetes, including lifestyle recommendations such as diet and exercise. The best doctors take a preventive approach to illness, rather than just treat the disease. They educate you about things like diet, exercise, and the importance of positive lifestyle changes.

Some red flags. Be wary of a doctor who hands you a list of foods and a "diabetic diet." Cookie-cutter approaches to diet are outmoded. In addition, you should be assigned to a registered dietitian who will customize a diet for you. Also, do not accept a doctor who shows no interest in your emotional health.

THE TEAM APPROACH: MAXIMIZE YOUR CHANCES OF GETTING THE BEST CARE

Your doctor will organize a team of health care professionals to help you with important aspects of self-care, as well as to check for and diagnose diabetic-related complications. In addition to your doctor, this team generally consists of the following:

Registered dietitian. Your dietitian helps you decide on a meal-planning system (see Step 1) that works best for you, plus teaches you how to plan your meals. Your dietitian can also design a weight-loss diet or a diet that restricts sodium or saturated fat. Make sure you go to a registered dietitian, designated by the initials RD. If the dietitian is a certified diabetes educator (CDE) (see below), all the better.

Diabetes educator. This professional may be a nurse or a dietitian and should have the initials CDE (certified diabetes educator) next to his or her title. A diabetes educator counsels you on various aspects of self-care, including following your diet, taking medications, testing your blood sugar, and handling stress and illnesses. A nurse CDE is often the main provider of care and education. You can locate a CDE by city and state through the Web site of the American Association of Diabetes Educators at www.aadenet.org.

Exercise physiologist. Regular exercise is a vital component in controlling diabetes, which is why you may want to work with an exercise physiologist, someone who has a university degree in exercise science. Further, he or she may be certified as an exercise trainer. An exercise physiologist can develop an exercise program suited for your particular situation and work with your doctor to ensure that you exercise safely.

Ophthalmologist. This is a medical doctor who specializes in the treatment of eye diseases. If you have eye problems, see an ophthalmologist who is familiar with diabetic eye disease.

Podiatrist. This health care professional is a foot doctor who treats foot injuries and problems such as calluses, sores, or ulcers. Look for someone who has experience in treating diabetic-related foot problems and who is a graduate from a college of podiatry with a doctor of podiatric medicine (DPM) degree.

Pharmacist. A pharmacist can provide a wealth of information about insulin or oral diabetes drugs, side effects of those drugs, nutritional supplements, and diabetes self-care products. As a general rule, you should get all your medications from the same pharmacy. That way the pharmacist can be on the lookout for drug interactions.

Dentist. With diabetes, your body has a tough time fighting off infections, including bacterial infections of the mouth and gums. Make sure you see a dentist every six months for a thorough oral examination and teeth cleaning. If you notice any unusual symptoms in your mouth, see your dentist right away.

Dermatologist. Because diabetes increases your risk of developing skin problems, it is important to have a qualified dermatologist on your team. A dermatologist is a medical doctor who specializes in the treatment of skin diseases. Find a dermatologist who understands diabetic-related skin problems.

Mental health therapist. There are various types of mental health professionals who can help you deal with the understandable anxiety and depression that often accompany a diagnosis of diabetes. These professionals include social workers, marriage and family therapists, clinical psychologists, and psychiatrists. With the exception of a psychiatrist (who has a medical degree), your therapist should have at least a master's degree in counseling and sufficient experience in counseling people with diabetes.

Alternative care practitioner. More than ever, people are turning to alternative medicine for disease prevention and treatment. A study published in the *Journal of the American Medical Association* reported that four out of every ten Americans are using alternative therapies. Alternative medicine includes such therapies as nutritional supplements, herbs, yoga, massage, hypnotherapy, and relaxation techniques and is provided by people who have special training and education in these areas. Increasingly, alternative medicine is being used as supportive treatment for diabetes. If you're considering or using alternative medicine, discuss its advisability with your physician.

Your insurance provider. In addition to having a qualified health care team, find out if your insurance company will cover everything you need for your diabetes treatment. Make sure your insurance plan provides you with the best care possible, including reimbursement for diabetes education, supplies, medications, alternative treatment, and the cost of specialists, if necessary.

If you're a member of an HMO, determine whether it is accredited by the National Committee of Quality Assurance (NCQA). The NCQA is an independent, not-for-profit organization dedicated to assessing and reporting on the quality of a variety of managed care plans. Its accreditation process evaluates how well a health plan manages all parts of its delivery system—physicians, hospitals, other providers and administrative service—in order to continuously improve health care for its members.

YOUR MEDICAL TEAM AND ROUTINE CARE

Once you're under the care of a great medical team, the next order of business is understanding the medical tests, medications, and routine care required to help you stay healthy and complication-free. That's the topic we'll turn to next.

Medical Tests and Medications That Can Save Your Life

Suppose you're having trouble with your vision. You chalk it up to a problem with your glasses or contact lenses. But could it be a sign of retinopathy?

Maybe you've lost your sexual desire on an occasion or two. Is it stress, or something more sinister, such as nerve damage?

Perhaps you've felt more dragged out than usual. You blame it on lack of sleep and vow to get more shut-eye next week. But could you be having heart or kidney trouble and just not know it?

In their early stages, the complications of diabetes often keep quiet until they become quite advanced and far more serious. Complications may be brewing, but you may never know it.

Is there a way to find out—and head them off at the pass?

Definitely: through regular physical examinations and laboratory tests. These are the tools your doctor and health care team use to detect signs of impending danger and prescribe corrective action to keep problems from developing into full-blown complications.

To help you stay complication-free, here's a look at what tests and examinations should be performed when you see your doctor at your initial visit and during follow-up visits.

THE INITIAL VISIT

If you're seeing a new doctor for the first time, the initial visit should have four parts:

Part 1: A detailed medical history taken by the doctor. This usually takes the form of an interview in which you're asked questions about the following:

- Existing symptoms
- Eating habits and diet
- Unusual weight gain or loss
- Previous and current treatment program
- Medicines and supplements you're taking
- Prior results of any blood sugar tests
- Exercise history
- Signs of complications, including vision problems, extreme fatigue, leg discomfort when walking, numbness or tingling in feet, chest pain upon exertion, long-to-heal sores or cuts, or frequent headaches
- History of infections, particularly skin, foot, dental, vaginal, and urinary tract infections
- Surgeries you've had
- Pregnancies
- Other medical problems you've had
- Family history of illness, including diabetes
- Risk factors for heart disease
- Tobacco and alcohol use

Part 2: A complete physical examination. Your doctor will:

- Measure your height and weight
- Take your blood pressure (see box on page 31 for an explanation of healthy blood pressure readings)
- Look in your eyes and refer you to an ophthalmologist for an eye exam
- Touch your neck to feel your thyroid gland and do tests if needed
- Listen to your heartbeat, heart rhythm, and lungs through a stethoscope
- Feel your abdomen to check your liver and other internal organs
- Take your pulse
- Check your feet, hands, and skin
- Test your reflexes
- Examine your gums and oral cavity

Part 3: Laboratory evaluation. This involves specific tests on your blood and urine to check your blood sugar level, the presence of ketones (by-products of fat metabolism that may indicate diabetes-related problems), your cholesterol and triglyceride levels (see box that follows), thyroid-stimulating hormone (for people with type 1 diabetes), serum creatinine (to check kidney function), and your urine protein level. It may also involve an electrocardiogram (EKG), treadmill stress test, or other tests, particularly if you plan to start an exercise program. (See the information on having a preparticipation physical on pages 50–54.)

Part 4: Establishment of a diabetes care plan that is tailored to

CHOLESTEROL AND TRIGLYCERIDE RISK LEVELS IN DIABETES			
BLOOD FAT	**LOW RISK**	**BORDERLINE RISK**	**HIGH RISK**
LDL	Less than 100 mg/dl	100–129 mg/dl	130 mg/dl or higher
HDL	More than 45 mg/dl (men); more than 55 mg/dl (women)	35–45 mg/dl (men); 45–55 mg/dl (women)	Less than 35 mg/dl (men); less than 45 mg/dl (women)
Triglycerides	Less than 200 mg/dl	200–399 mg/dl	400 mg/dl or higher

This chart illustrates the various risk levels for people with diabetes. Like blood glucose, your cholesterol and triglycerides are measured in milligrams per deciliter of blood (mg/dl). Your cholesterol and triglyceride counts are used to predict your risk of developing cardiovascular disease.

Source: D'Arrigo, T. 1999. Cholesterol: The good, the bad, and the ugly. *Diabetes Forecast*, October 1, pp. 54–58.

your own life, work schedule, activity level, foods you like, cultural background, and existing medical problems. Your diabetes care plan should include:

- A list of short- and long-term goals
- A list of medications you will take to control your diabetes, particularly if you have type 1 diabetes (not all people with type 2 diabetes take medications)
- Choice of a meal-planning system and how to use it (a dietitian should be assigned to help you with this)
- A list of lifestyle changes you must make, such as getting more exercise or quitting smoking
- Instructions on how to monitor your blood sugar levels and test urine ketone levels

- A schedule of instructional sessions for you and your family on how to measure your blood sugar levels and ketones, how to keep records, and how to treat hypoglycemia
- An annual referral to an ophthalmologist, podiatrist, dentist, and other specialists, if needed
- Instructions on continuing care

FUTURE VISITS AND CONTINUING CARE

Regular follow-up visits throughout the year are vital for controlling your diabetes. How often you visit your doctor depends on many factors. For example, if you're meeting your goals and controlling your blood sugar, you may need to see your doctor only once or twice a year. On the other hand, if you're not meeting your goals, you may have to schedule more frequent appointments. Patients taking insulin or being switched to new diabetes medications may have to visit their doctors more often too. Of course, if you get sick or experience any unusual symptoms, you should see your doctor right away.

During follow-up visits, your physician will order a *glycohemoglobin test*. Also referred to as a glycated or glycosylated hemoglobin test, this test measures the concentration of hemoglobin molecules in your red blood cells to determine the percentage of molecules that are *glycated*, that is, have glucose attached to them. A 9 percent reading means that 9 percent of your hemoglobin is glycated. Nondiabetics have about a 5 percent level. A high GHb (9 percent or above) is considered a risk factor for diabetes complications. Your goal should be less than 7 percent. If your test results exceed 8 percent, your physician will make adjustments in your treatment plan.

The more glucose you have in your blood, the more hemoglobin will become glycated. Once hemoglobin becomes glycated, it stays that way throughout the life span of the red blood cell, which is about three months. The GHb test can thus tell your doctor what your average blood glucose level has been over the past three months.

Worth noting is that glycation produces *advanced glycated end products* (AGEs), which are among the substances that can damage tissues, leading to diabetic complications. There are natural remedies to minimize the formation of these toxic substances. You'll learn more about these remedies in Step 2.

There are several types of GHb tests. The most common are HbA1C and HbA1. HbA1C is a very specific test that measures the hemoglobin-glucose linkage at only one site on the hemoglobin molecule. HbA1 is simply another form of glycohemoglobin that is measured. No GHb test is better than another. All forms of glycohemoglobin tests provide the same useful data about your average blood glucose levels.

The GHb test is not used to diagnose diabetes, because some people with the disease can have normal GHb levels. Instead, the test is used to monitor blood glucose control and the effectiveness of diabetic treatments, plus help people with diabetes better manage the disease. Generally, your doctor will check your GHb levels at regular intervals: twice a year if stable, or quarterly if you're not meeting your goals.

During follow-up visits, your doctor will also:

- Ask you about times you've experienced high or low blood sugar
- Review records you've kept on your blood sugar levels
- Ask if you've had trouble sticking to your diabetes care plan
- Ask about symptoms that may indicate diabetic complications

- Ask about medical problems or recent illnesses
- Ask about the results of dental exams, eye tests, or tests conducted by other specialists
- Measure your weight and blood pressure
- Check your feet (annually)
- Review and adjust medication
- Review your diet and exercise activities
- Ask about tobacco and alcohol use
- Order a fasting lipid profile (to check your cholesterol and triglycerides), serum creatinine, and a urinalysis (usually done annually)
- Ask about your emotional health and adjustment to diabetes
- Evaluate your diabetes care plan to assess your progress in meeting goals and to identify problem areas

The tests and exams you need on a periodic basis are summarized in the box opposite, according to which type of diabetes you have.

YOUR EXERCISE PLAN: THE PREPARTICIPATION EVALUATION

Starting an exercise program is one of the best ways to manage your diabetes, plus improve your sense of well-being and overall quality of life. But before you jump into a jogging suit or head to the gym, consult your physician to undergo a preparticipation evaluation. This is a special medical examination that rules out any health problems that could keep you from exercising. It assesses the health status of your heart, chest, and lungs; the strength of various body parts; joint mobility; the condition of other body parts and organs; your weight; and your percentage of body fat and

YOUR SCHEDULE FOR KEY TESTS AND EXAMS

TESTS AND EXAMS	TYPE 1 DIABETES	TYPE 2 DIABETES
General physical exam	Once a year	Once a year
Blood and urine tests to check for kidney disease	Once a year	Once a year
Glycohemoglobin (GHb) tests	4 times a year	Twice a year; 4 times a year if diabetes is poorly controlled
Dilated eye exam by an ophthalmologist	Once a year	Once a year
Lipid profile (cholesterol and triglycerides)	Once a year, or as recommended by your doctor; every 3 to 6 months if levels are abnormal	Once a year, or as recommended by your doctor; every 3 to 6 months if levels are abnormal
Checkups for specific problems (impotence, numbness, tingling, stomach distress, swelling, blurred vision, chest pain, foot infections)	As soon as the problem occurs	As soon as the problem occurs
Blood pressure	At every doctor visit	At every doctor visit
Foot exam	At every doctor visit	At every doctor visit
Dental exam	Every 6 months	Every 6 months

muscle. A blood test may be administered in order to double-check your cholesterol and triglyceride levels.

Because you have diabetes, your physician will evaluate your glucose control and discuss your use of prescribed medications. Your preparticipation evaluation will also zero in on symptoms of medical conditions affecting the cardiovascular system, eyes, kidneys, and nervous system, provided they haven't been examined in previous medical checkups.

The evaluation helps pinpoint which exercises you must avoid, particularly if your doctor finds any medical complications or physical limitations. If everything looks good, you'll be given the go-ahead to exercise. But if your doctor finds complications, you may be advised to forgo exercise until these problems are treated or resolved.

Cardiovascular and Circulatory Status

To check for underlying heart and blood vessel problems, you should have a stress test with EKG monitoring. Identifying any type of abnormality—or simply verifying that you're fit—can make you a more effective exerciser and a healthier person overall.

With diabetes, circulation to the legs and feet is often sluggish. About one-third of older people with diabetes have poor circulation to the extremities.

Your physician will check for symptoms of circulatory problems, which include cold feet, pain, decreased or absent pulse, and loss of tissue in the extremities. Decreased circulation can result in complications such as intermittent claudification (leg pain and cramps), loss of nerve tissue and sensitivity in the feet, foot infections, and gangrene.

If your circulation is impaired, you may be instructed to avoid any exercise that places undue strain on your feet, such as jogging, walking, or aerobic dancing. Better choices include non-weight-bearing activities such as swimming, water exercise, or stationary cycling. In addition, you must learn how to take care of your feet during a workout, including the selection of proper footwear. Always inspect your feet and toes daily for sores, cuts, swelling, cold areas (a sign of poor circulation), and warm areas (a sign of infection).

Assessment of Retinopathy

Before beginning an exercise program, be sure to have an eye examination performed by an ophthalmologist. Anyone who has or is at extreme risk of developing diabetic retinopathy will have to select nonjarring, nonstraining exercises such as swimming or stationary cycling instead of jogging, playing racquet sports, or lifting weights. The latter activities increase your risk of eye hemorrhage or retinal detachment.

Assessment of Nephropathy

An early sign of nephropathy (kidney disease) is small amounts of protein in your urine (microalbuminuria). Your physician will check for this on a regular basis. It can be managed with good glucose control, a low-salt diet, and blood pressure medicine.

If you have or are at risk of developing nephropathy, your physician will probably discourage you from performing high-effort or strenuous exercises such as running, aerobic dancing, or strength training. These forms of exercise can elevate your systolic blood pressure (the top number in a blood pressure reading), aggravating existing kidney disease. Lower-intensity activities such as walking are preferred for patients with nephropathy.

Assessment of Neuropathy

Patients with diabetes often experience various types of neuropathy (nerve disease). Distal symmetric neuropathy and focal neuropathy, which accompany impaired circulation, involve a loss of nerve tissue and sensitivity in the extremities, particularly the feet and legs. They may feel numb, as if they've "gone to sleep." Sores may develop and, if untreated, may become infected.

To check for these types of neuropathy, your physician will test your reflexes, sense of touch, and ability to feel pain, heat, and cold. Other neurological tests may be performed as well.

If you have lost sensation in your feet, you'll be advised to avoid exercises such as prolonged walking, treadmill exercise, jogging, or step aerobics. Better choices include swimming, bicycling, rowing, chair exercises, arm exercises, and any non-weight-bearing activity. Always wear proper footwear (including socks), regardless of the activity.

Autonomic neuropathy damages nerves in the body that control involuntary actions such as heartbeat and respiration. Your physician looks for signs of autonomic neuropathy by listening to your heart and lungs, monitoring your resting heart rate, taking blood pressure, and checking for abnormalities involving your skin, pupils, digestive system, or urinary system.

Autonomic neuropathy causes high or low blood pressure and can abnormally increase heart rate. Thus, anyone who has or is at risk of this complication should pursue nonstrenuous, easy-does-it exercises such as slow walking, which will not spike blood pressure or overly accelerate the heart rate.

Autonomic neuropathy also affects your ability to sense hot or cold temperatures. Thus, you should not exercise in extremes of weather.

GO FOR IT

By learning from your doctor what you can and cannot do, the odds are that your exercise program will bring nothing but healthy rewards—plus step up the quality of your life.

IF YOU HAVE TO TAKE DIABETES MEDICATIONS

Depending on your situation, your doctor may prescribe medication to treat your diabetes: self-administered insulin or oral diabetes medications (if you have type 2 diabetes). During office visits, your doctor will explain how to use these medications and conduct periodic blood tests to gauge how your body is responding to treatment. You'll learn more about how to use these medications in Step 5. For now, here's some important background on the medications used to treat diabetes.

INSULIN

If you have type 1 diabetes, your body does not produce any or enough insulin, and therefore you must depend on supplemental insulin to survive. On the other hand, people with type 2 diabetes do not depend on insulin, but over time their insulin production may decrease. This necessitates the use of self-administered insulin for adequate blood glucose control, particularly during times of stress or illness. In type 2 diabetes, self-administered insulin is often recommended if your glycated hemoglobin stays over 8 percent, despite the use of oral diabetes medications. In all cases of insulin therapy, your dosage must be individualized and balanced with diet and exercise.

Self-administered insulin is obtained from a genetically engineered process in which bacteria or yeast are turned into little production centers that make synthetic human insulin. In the past, the most commonly used insulins were produced from pork, beef, or pork-beef combinations. Animal-source insulins, however, can cause allergic reactions and have been or are being discontinued because of the wide availability of synthetic human insulins. Still, many people have used animal-source insulin for years without any problems. For people newly diagnosed with diabetes, the American Diabetes Association recommends the use of human insulin, which is absorbed more quickly than other forms are.

If your doctor prescribes insulin, it is important to understand the various types of insulin and how they work. This information is discussed below; however, be sure to have your doctor thoroughly explain insulin treatment to you. Take notes, and ask questions if you don't understand something.

Types of Insulin

Self-administered insulin has four basic characteristics, which are important for understanding how it acts medicinally to control blood glucose.

Onset is the length of time it takes insulin to reach your bloodstream and start reducing your blood glucose levels.

Peak time refers to the period during which insulin is at its highest strength in terms of reducing blood glucose levels.

Duration describes how long insulin continues to work to lower blood glucose levels.

Strength is the concentration of insulin in a preparation. Most insulin preparations sold in the United States have the same strength: U-100. This means they have 100 units of insulin in every cubic centimeter (cc) of fluid. There are preparations of U-500, but these are for special cases in which patients need extremely high doses, or for use by hospitals for emergencies.

There are several major types of insulin. Each is designed for different situations and lifestyles. Your doctor will decide which ones are best for you, based on your personal situation and how you respond to insulin. The box on page 58 provides a brief rundown of the various types of insulin available and how they work.

Premixed Insulins

Most people with diabetes use insulin mixtures. Basically, these are combinations of intermediate and regular-acting insulin in one syringe. You may have to mix the insulins yourself or purchase them already mixed.

ORAL MEDICINES FOR TYPE 2 DIABETES

Your physician may prescribe oral diabetes medications to help lower your blood sugar and get your diabetes under control. This decision is usually made when tests show that your blood glucose levels are not adequately controlled by diet, exercise, and weight loss:

- Your blood glucose levels before breakfast exceed 140 mg/dl.
- Your blood glucose levels before bedtime exceed 160 mg/dl; or
- Your glycohemoglobin test exceeds 8 percent

Taking these medications, however, does not mean that you can forget about eating sensibly and exercising regularly. Oral diabetes medications, also known as oral hypoglycemic agents, are designed to work with your meal plan and exercise program.

Oral medications are not insulin. Nor are they meant for people with type 1 diabetes, because the pancreas doesn't manufacture

CHARACTERISTICS AND ACTIONS OF INSULIN

TYPE	ONSET	PEAK	DURATION	SOURCE*	SPECIAL CONSIDERATIONS
Rapid-acting (lispro)	Within 5 minutes after injection	Within 60 minutes after injection	2–4 hours	Human	• Injected immediately before a meal • Maintains blood glucose levels below 180 mg/dl for 2 hours after eating
Regular or short-acting	30 minutes after injection	2–3 hours after injection	3–6 hours	Human or animal (pork or beef)	• The most reliably absorbed insulin
Intermediate-acting (NPH or Lente)	2–4 hours after injection	4–12 hours after injection	12–18 hours	Human or animal (pork or beef)	• Often used in combination with short-acting insulin
Long-acting	6–10 hours after injection	14–24 hours after injection	20–36 hours	Human	• Provides a nearly continuous release of insulin • Often combined with a short-acting insulin • Recommended at bedtime to maintain blood sugar control overnight
Ultralente	Absorbed at different rates in different people	8–10 or 12–16 hours after injection	20–24 hours	Human	• Usually administered twice a day or once a day, usually at bedtime

CHARACTERISTICS AND ACTIONS OF INSULIN (cont'd)					
TYPE	ONSET	PEAK	DURATION	SOURCE*	SPECIAL CONSIDERATIONS
Glargine (Lantus)	Rapid	Peakless action because it mimics the body's natural insulin secretion	Around the clock with just one injection	Human	• Must not be mixed with other types of insulin

Source: Adapted from Insulin. *Diabetes Forecast 2001 Buyer's Guide*, p. 46; Hirsch, I. B. 1999. Type 1 diabetes mellitus and the use of flexible insulin regimens. *American Family Physician*, November 15.

*The source of insulin affects how rapidly insulin is absorbed, peaks, and lasts. Human-source insulins are absorbed faster than other forms.

enough insulin for the pills to do any good. For people with type 1 diabetes, insulin therapy is the only way to reduce blood glucose levels.

In general, oral diabetes medications work in one or more of the following ways:

- Help your pancreas release more insulin
- Stimulate your body's ability to use the insulin it produces
- Reduce the amount of glucose produced by your liver
- Slow or block the absorption of starches and sugars from food

Sometimes, oral diabetes pills stop working after a few months or a few years. No one has yet pinpointed exactly why this happens, but it doesn't mean your diabetes has gotten worse. If your diabetes pill stops working, switching to another drug won't solve the problem. Instead, your physician may add another oral diabetes agent to your therapy.

If your oral medicine does its job, you may still need to take insulin if you get sick or need surgery. The reason is that pills may not work as well during stressful times when blood glucose tends to soar. If you are planning to become pregnant, you'll need to stop taking diabetes pills and switch to insulin until your baby is born. (Taking insulin while breast-feeding is fine, however.) Your physician will advise you on what to do.

All oral diabetes medications interact with a variety of other drugs, so you should tell your physician and pharmacist about *all* drugs you're taking, including over-the-counter medicines. Understanding how your oral medication works will help you use it properly for the best results.

Now let's talk about another kind of "medicine" that will work wonders in controlling your diabetes—and do it naturally: good nutrition.

Eat to Beat Diabetes: Understanding the Role of Nutrition

Food is one of the chief tools you can use to control your diabetes and stay healthy. It helps keep your blood sugar in line, provides energy for exercise and daily activities, and supplies the nutrients needed for health and healing. Food is nourishment and medicine all rolled into one.

What kind of food should you eat? A prevailing myth about diabetes is that you must follow a special "diabetic diet." Not so. You have the same nutritional needs as anyone else. Like the rest of the world, you need regular, well-balanced meals that provide a variety of nutrients. Those nutrients come from five major food groups: carbohydrates, protein, fats, vitamins, and minerals.

CARBOHYDRATES

Plentiful in grains, cereal, breads, pasta, vegetables, and fruits, carbohydrates are to your body what gas is to a car—the fuel that gets you going. In fact, the major role of carbohydrates is to provide energy.

For people with diabetes, carbohydrates are very important, since they have the most pronounced effect on blood glucose levels. During digestion, carbohydrates are broken down into molecules of glucose. Assisted by insulin, glucose is directed into cells to be used by various tissues in the body.

Several things can happen to glucose. Once inside a cell, it can be quickly metabolized to supply energy. Or it may be converted to either liver or muscle glycogen, the storage form of carbohydrate. When you exercise or use your muscles, the body mobilizes muscle glycogen for energy. Blood glucose can also turn into body fat and get packed away in fat tissue. This happens when you eat more carbohydrates than you need or than your body can store as liver or muscle glycogen. Some blood glucose may also be excreted in the urine.

There are two classes of carbohydrates: complex carbohydrates and simple carbohydrates. Complex carbohydrates, also called *starches*, include most plant foods: cereals, pasta, fruits, and vegetables. They're packed with vitamins and minerals, not to mention fiber, an indigestible carbohydrate that is vital in diabetic nutrition. Fiber helps reduce blood sugar levels and protect against heart disease.

Simple carbohydrates, otherwise known as *simple sugars*, include glucose, fructose, galactose, sucrose, and lactose. Glucose and fructose are found mostly in fruits; galactose and lactose are sugars in milk. Sucrose is found in ordinary table sugar. Candy, desserts, baked goods, and other processed foods tend to be high in simple sugars.

In a diet designed to control diabetes, it's preferable to emphasize complex carbohydrates and downplay simple sugars. Simple sugars are a major source of calories but offer no nutrients to go along with the calories. Because of this, it's best to limit simple sugars in your diet.

PROTEIN

You need protein from food to support the growth and maintenance of your body. The protein you eat is broken down into tiny fragments called amino acids. These are used to manufacture muscle and other tissues; hemoglobin, which carries oxygen to cells; enzymes and hormones, which regulate all body processes; and antibodies, which fight off infection and disease. Amino acids also form DNA and RNA, special proteins inside cells that control cellular growth and reproduction, thus governing all life.

Protein is available from most foods, but is highest in meat, fish, eggs, and dairy products. Certain vegetables are high in protein as well, especially legumes such as soybeans, kidney beans, lentils, and lima beans. Nuts and seeds are rich in protein too.

Protein helps stabilize blood sugar. By combining protein, complex carbohydrates, and fat in the same meal, you automatically slow-release glucose because your digestive system takes longer to break down this combination of foods. This manner of food combining helps prevent spikes in blood sugar after eating.

FATS

Controlling diabetes means controlling the amount and type of fat in your diet. Too much of the wrong type of fat can lead to heart disease and other cardiovascular complications. Your diet must supply some fat, however, because fat helps slow your digestion to prevent spikes in blood sugar following a meal.

Most dietary fats are technically known as *triglycerides*. During digestion, triglycerides are broken down into fatty acids and absorbed into the cells of the intestinal walls. The stored fat in your body is also made up of mostly triglycerides.

Another classification of fat is the *sterols*. The best-known sterol is *cholesterol*, an odorless, waxy, fatlike substance found in all foods of animal origin. Needed for good health, cholesterol is a constituent of most body tissues. It is also used to make certain hormones, vitamin D, and bile. If your body churns out too much cholesterol, the excess circulates in the bloodstream and collects in the inner walls of the arteries—a condition that can lead to a heart attack.

The type of cholesterol responsible for depositing cholesterol in the artery walls is low-density lipoprotein, or LDL cholesterol. LDLs are known as the "bad" cholesterol. Bad cholesterol comes in another form called very-low-density lipoprotein (VLDL), and scientists believe that this type is more harmful to your cardiovascular system than LDL cholesterol is.

By contrast, high-density lipoprotein, or HDL cholesterol, is heart-protective. Its job is to remove bad cholesterol from the cells in the artery wall and transport it back to the liver for reprocessing or excretion from the body as waste. HDL is "good" cholesterol; the more in your blood, the better.

Dietary fats are either *saturated* or *unsaturated*—terms that describe their chemical structure. Saturated fats are found mostly in beef, dairy products, commercially prepared baked goods, and tropical oils like coconut, palm, and palm kernel oils. These fats can promote insulin resistance and glucose intolerance. What's more, they can raise LDL cholesterol to potentially dangerous levels.

Unsaturated fats aren't quite as harmful. In fact, they contain key nutrients called essential fatty acids. Two of the most important are linoleic acid, found in vegetable oils, and linolenic acid, found in fish. Essential fatty acids are required for normal growth, skin integrity, and healthy blood and nerves.

There are two categories of unsaturated fats: *polyunsaturated fats* and *monounsaturated fats*. Vegetable oils such as safflower oil, sunflower oil, corn oil, soybean oil, and cottonseed oil are polyunsaturated fats.

A special group of polyunsaturated fat is the omega-3 fatty acids, abundant in fish. They protect against the development of glucose intolerance. Along with omega-6 fatty acids (found mostly in vegetable oils), omega-3 fats are now considered essential fats that must be included in your diet.

Monounsaturated fats have a protective effect on blood cholesterol levels. They help lower the bad cholesterol but maintain higher levels of the good cholesterol. They also help keep blood pressure in check and reduce levels of triglycerides in the blood. Monounsaturated fats are plentiful in olive oil, canola oil, and peanut oil, and in fish from cold waters, such as salmon, mackerel, halibut, swordfish, black cod, and rainbow trout, and in shellfish.

As for other dietary fats, watch out for foods containing *trans-fatty acids*. These are produced when vegetable oils are altered chemically through a process called hydrogenation, in which hydrogen is forced into the oil to make it harder and more spreadable. Some margarines and numerous processed foods such as fast foods, crackers, chips, and baked goods are high in trans-fatty acids. These commercially processed unsaturated fats behave more like saturated fats. Research indicates that hydrogenated fats and the trans-fatty acids they contain may elevate LDL cholesterol and lower beneficial HDL cholesterol.

VITAMINS AND MINERALS

Provided by foods and supplements, vitamins and minerals are involved in regulating digestion, muscle contraction, growth and repair, wound healing, metabolism, and other life-giving processes.

Many minerals provide the structural strength for your bones and other tissues.

People with diabetes are often deficient in many vitamins and minerals. That's why it's vital to eat a variety of foods, including vegetables, fruits, whole grains, protein foods, and dairy products. As additional insurance, it's a good idea to supplement your diet with vitamins and minerals.

A standard called the Daily Reference Intake (DRI) is a new way of rating the amounts of the vitamins, minerals, and protein we need for good health and the prevention of chronic disease. The DRI contains four different rating sets: the familiar recommended daily allowance (RDA), which designates amounts of nutrients that maintain health; the estimated average requirement, which describes the daily requirement needed for 50 percent of Americans; tolerable upper intake levels, which establish ceilings to help us avoid taking too much of a nutrient; and adequate intakes, which is an estimate of average intake that seems healthy and won't harm health. For the purposes of this book, nutrient recommendations are placed under the heading of DRIs. In Step 2, "Drive Diabetes into Retreat with Natural Remedies," you'll learn more about specific vitamins and minerals that are helpful in treating diabetes and preventing its complications.

FROM SUGAR TO ALCOHOL: ARE THERE FORBIDDEN FOODS IN DIABETES THERAPY?

There's a lot of confusion about what people with diabetes can and cannot eat. Actually, very few foods are off-limits. Still, some foods should be deemphasized in your diet: sugar and certain sweeteners, sodium, caffeine, and alcohol. Here's a rundown of what you need to know.

Sugar and Sweeteners

For nearly one hundred years, people with diabetes were told to shun sugar. It was believed that sugar would send glucose levels soaring. But research shows otherwise. Eating sugar and sugar-containing foods does not interfere with glucose control in either type 1 or type 2 diabetes. It is perfectly fine to substitute sugar and sugar-containing foods for other carbohydrates in your diet. You don't really have to avoid table sugar, corn sweeteners, syrups, or other such foods.

However, don't go overboard. Sugar has no nutrients, so it should be restricted in your diet. Too much sugar has been associated with tooth decay, obesity, and cardiovascular disease.

If you wish to limit sugar, satisfy your sweet tooth with fruit, which is loaded with health-building nutrients. Or opt for artificial sweeteners, particularly if you are trying to lose weight. Artificial sweeteners include saccharin, aspartame, and acesulfame K, which are approved for use by the FDA. Still, these sweeteners have been linked to adverse health effects.

That being so, you might want to consider a natural sweetener called stevia, derived from the *Stevia rebaudiana* shrub grown in South America. Its leaves yield a sugarlike derivative called steviocide, which is 250 to 300 times sweeter than sugar and is noncaloric.

Stevia has been a popular sweetener in Japan for more than twenty years. What's more, it has long been used in Paraguay and Brazil to treat diabetes. A recent animal study found that two active ingredients in stevia—steviocide and steviol—stimulated insulin secretion by acting directly on beta cells.

Available as tea, powdered leaves, a liquid extract, and purified steviocide, the herb is considered a dietary supplement in the United States by Food and Drug Administration definition. Stevia has not yet been granted safe status as a food additive by the FDA and technically cannot be labeled as a sweetener.

Even so, you can sweeten foods with stevia, as well as bake with it. The trick is to use minute amounts, because the more stevia you use, the more bitter it tastes. Barely a pinch will sweeten your coffee or herbal tea, and one shake on a bowl of cereal imparts just enough sweet taste. For baking, one teaspoon of stevia extract is the equivalent of one cup of sugar. You'll have to experiment to achieve the desired sweetness.

Other sweeteners include sugar alcohols, such as mannitol, sorbitol, xylitol, and maltitol, which are found mostly in low-calorie food products. All four contain roughly the same number of calories as sugar (3 to 4 calories per gram). So if you're trying to cut calories, sugar alcohols offer little benefit. However, these sweeteners are more slowly absorbed than sugar is. For this reason, the sugar alcohols are thought to be better than sugar for people with diabetes who are trying to keep blood glucose at healthy levels.

Sodium

Your body depends on sodium to help regulate the amount of fluid that surrounds cells. In the diet, sodium is obtained mostly from salt and processed foods. Recommendations for sodium intake for people with diabetes are the same as for the general public. You should consume less than 2,400 milligrams a day, or no more than 1¼ teaspoons of table salt. If you have high blood pressure or kidney disease, a healthier target is less than 2,000 milligrams daily. The minimum requirement for adults is 500 milligrams a day, an amount provided by eating plain foods with no salt added. Many people with diabetes are overly sensitive to salt, so you may want to shoot for the minimum.

One of the best ways to cut down on sodium intake is to avoid processed, snack, and fast foods, which contribute as much as 75 percent of the salt consumed in our diets. Other ways to reduce intake are to cook with only small amounts of salt and to season foods with sodium-free spices.

Caffeine

You know caffeine best as the ingredient in your coffee and tea that gets you going in the morning, but it is also a drug—in fact, it is the most widely used drug in the world. That being the case, is it a good idea to use caffeine if your goal is to control your diabetes and improve your health?

In moderate amounts, caffeine and beverages containing it are probably not harmful. However, caffeine may aggravate certain health problems, such as heart disease and high blood pressure—both of which are complications of diabetes. If you have such complications, you may want to cut out the caffeine for the sake of your long-term health.

Alcohol

Can you still enjoy a cocktail or two, considering you have diabetes? The answer is a guarded yes, as long as you understand some ground rules. You can consume alcohol in moderation (no more than two drinks a day if you're a man and no more than one drink a day if you're a woman, provided:

- Your diabetes is well controlled. (Moderate alcohol use usually doesn't affect blood glucose levels when diabetes is under control.)
- Your physician confirms that you have no health problems, such as diabetic nerve damage or high blood pressure.
- You understand how alcohol consumption affects you and your diabetes.

Alcohol is essentially a toxin, and your body treats it as such. Alcohol requires no digestion and rushes to your brain within a minute. About thirty to ninety minutes later, it reaches peak levels in your bloodstream.

One of the risks involved in drinking alcohol is the possibility of low blood sugar. Here's why: Normally, when your blood sugar dips, your liver starts converting stored carbohydrate (glycogen) into glucose, which is then dispatched into the bloodstream. This counteracts low blood sugar.

But when alcohol is in your body, things change. Because alcohol is a toxin, disposing of it becomes your liver's top priority. The liver won't even start converting glycogen into glucose until it has done away with the alcohol. So if your blood sugar starts to fall and you're drinking alcohol, you could experience hypoglycemia very quickly. To avoid this reaction, never drink alcohol on an empty stomach, but always with meals or snacks.

If you've enjoyed an evening of cocktails, have a snack before bedtime to prevent a hypoglycemic reaction while you're asleep.

Keep in mind, too, that the body treats alcohol like a fat. Alcohol is ultimately converted into fatty acids and thus is more likely to be stored as body fat. Drinking alcohol is not a wise decision if you're trying to lose weight.

Excessive alcohol intake increases your odds of developing heart disease, a complication of diabetes. More than two drinks a day can raise your blood pressure and contribute to high triglycerides, a risk factor for heart disease. Drinking large amounts of alcohol regularly can also cause heart failure and lead to stroke.

Finally, alcohol is a depressant. If you suffer from depression—many people with diabetes do—you should skip alcohol.

Diabetic Foods

There are special foods marketed for people with diabetes. However, many diabetes experts advise against their use. Writing in the *British Journal of Nursing,* Gillian Aitken put it this way: "Diabetic foods are not recommended. They are expensive and perpetuate the myth that a special diet is necessary."

The reasons diabetic foods get such low marks is that they are often higher in fat and sweeteners such as sorbitol, which can have a laxative effect if eaten in excess. Therefore, you don't need specially formulated foods in your diet. Stick to natural foods, which are packed with vitamins, minerals, fiber, and other vital nutrients.

BEYOND NUTRITION

There's no question that nutrition is an excellent way to redirect the course of diabetes. Doubling up with diet to keep blood sugar at near-normal levels is exercise, quite possibly the best "medicine" ever devised to fight diabetes. The benefits of exercise are discussed next.

The Exercise Connection

If you could bottle the benefits of exercise, it would be the single most prescribed diabetic medication in the world. That's because exercise helps you manage a life-and-death matter in diabetes: controlling your blood sugar, particularly in type 2 diabetes.

In effect, exercise normalizes blood sugar levels by making cells more sensitive to the action of insulin. Scientists aren't yet sure exactly how this happens, but there are some possible explanations. Exercise may increase the number of receptors on the outer surface of cells, thus making cells less resistant to insulin. Or exercise may bring about changes inside cells that allow more glucose to enter and provide fuel. What scientists do know is that muscles use more glucose during exercise, as much as seven to twenty times more than normal.

Whatever the precise mechanism may be, exercise performs a metabolic minimiracle by removing some glucose from blood to use for energy and thus reducing and controlling blood glucose levels. For people with type 1 diabetes, exercise often reduces the amount of supplemental insulin needed. Likewise, exercisers with type 2 diabetes may be able to reduce their dosage of medication.

Vitally important: Exercise helps deter and stop life-threatening complications of diabetes, such as heart disease, stroke, high blood pressure, eye trouble, nerve damage, and kidney disease.

Diabetes experts recommend that people with diabetes, who have no significant complications or limitations, follow a workout program that incorporates two types of exercise: aerobic exercise and strength training. Aerobic exercise is sustained activity that gets your heart pumping. It produces positive changes in the health of your heart and circulatory system. Aerobic exercise includes walking, treadmill walking, jogging, running, cross-country skiing, swimming, bicycling, and aerobic dancing.

Strength training—also called resistance training or weight training—is any kind of weight-bearing activity in which your muscles are challenged to work harder each time they're exercised. The purpose of strength training is to develop and preserve muscle. Examples of strength training are lifting weights, working out on weight-training machines, performing calisthenics, and exercising with special rubber bands or cords.

A combination of both forms of exercise controls your blood sugar, plus improves other health variables such as weight, blood pressure, and cholesterol. The remarkable benefits of combination exercise can stretch out your healthy life span for many years.

What follows is a closer look at the many powerful benefits you'll reap from each type of exercise.

AEROBIC EXERCISE: A POWERFUL PUNCH AGAINST DIABETES

Barring any medical complications or limitations, aerobic exercise can be safely performed if you have type 1 or type 2 diabetes. It is among the most effective ways to manage diabetes, plus steer you away from the troubling complications of the disease. In addition to its amazing ability to keep blood glucose in check, here are several specific benefits of aerobic exercise.

Fights Fat

The leading risk factor for getting type 2 diabetes is obesity—nearly 80 percent of all type 2 diabetics are overweight. But the encouraging news is that aerobic exercise is one of the best ways to achieve permanent weight loss and, in doing so, get your diabetes under control.

When you exercise aerobically, your body draws on fat in the form of fatty acids as one of its energy sources. Aerobic exercise also increases fat-burning enzymes in your body. You need those enzymes if you want to get fashionably fit. What's more, aerobic exercise builds your oxygen-processing capacity. Fat is burned only when there's adequate oxygen around. Finally, exercise bumps up your metabolism, which means your body becomes more efficient at burning calories, even at rest.

Losing weight through a combination of aerobics and calorie-controlled dieting significantly improves glucose control, according to studies of people with type 2 diabetes. And, if you've been taking diabetes medication, exercise and the weight loss it produces may enable you to decrease your medication.

Improves Heart Health

Heart disease is a life-threatening complication of type 1 and type 2 diabetes and the leading cause of death among diabetics. Fortunately, though, many studies have proved that aerobic exercise is an effective risk reducer for heart disease. An aerobically fit heart can pump more blood with each beat, during exercise and while at rest. Your heart rate slows too, so that when you climb a flight of stairs or play a set of tennis, your heart doesn't have to work as hard. You can be more active without running out of breath.

Your entire circulatory system changes too. Aerobic exercise makes your capillaries increase in size and number, so that more blood finds its way to the muscles and other tissues where it's needed. That's important to circulatory health, since many people with diabetes often develop blood vessel disease and impaired circulation.

Another reward of aerobic exercise is that it helps reduce the buildup of artery-clogging LDL cholesterol in your body.

Reduces High Blood Pressure

People with diabetes are at risk of developing high blood pressure, which ultimately damages your heart, blood vessels, and kidneys. One proven way to lower blood pressure is with aerobic exercise. Most studies of hypertensive people show that a reduction can occur with as little as three exercise sessions a week for thirty to sixty minutes each time. Exercise can prevent high blood pressure too.

Promotes Normal Blood Clotting

In many people with type 2 diabetes, the body is unable to dissolve blood clots in a normal fashion. As a result, tiny clotting elements in the blood called platelets tend to stick together when they're not supposed to. This can contribute to heart attack, stroke, and tiny eye hemorrhages. Aerobic exercise, however, has been shown to make platelets less sticky and thus normalize the blood-clotting process.

Brightens Your Mental Outlook

With diabetes, there is understandable stress, anxiety, and depression associated with the disease. Aerobic exercise, however, is one of the most effective ways to dissipate these negative emotions. It speeds up the production of feel-good endorphins, thought to be responsible for the pleasurable sensation called the "runner's high" that joggers and marathoners experience. The result is a general sense of mental well-being.

Exercise also relieves muscular tension brought on by stress and anxiety. In fact, numerous studies have shown that aerobic exercise can be an effective part of treatment for depression and anxiety. Further, the more you make exercise a habit, the better your mood and the lower your stress level.

STRENGTH TRAINING: EXERCISE CHAMPION

Strength training, which can be performed if you have type 1 or type 2 diabetes, offers numerous health-building advantages too.

Controls Blood Sugar

Strength training helps normalize the flow of glucose from the blood into the muscle tissue, where it can be properly used for energy. This effect may help regulate the body's use of glucose, thereby controlling or preventing diabetes and its complications.

Another plus for strength training: It reduces glycated hemoglobin in your blood. In one study, ten weeks of strength training decreased glycated hemoglobin immediately following exercise sessions. The process of glycation—the binding of glucose to hemoglobin or other substances—is damaging to the body over time. With the findings of the study as proof, it appears that strength training may help counteract this process.

Improves Insulin Action

Exercise encourages insulin use by activating a key protein in muscle cells that helps insulin push glucose into these cells. As noted earlier, muscle cells need lots of glucose for energy and therefore must rely heavily on insulin to get it.

Controls Weight

Strength training helps you get rid of unwanted fat by developing lean muscle. Firm, strong muscles are "metabolically active." This means they can burn body fat more efficiently than untoned muscle, even at rest. The more muscle you have, the more fat you can burn. In fact, it has been estimated that if you put on just five pounds of muscle, you'll burn between 50,000 and 90,000 more calories in one year! (That's a loss of fifteen to twenty-five pounds.) Lack of muscle, on the other hand, makes it easy for you to pack on fat pounds.

Reduces Blood Fats

There is overwhelming scientific proof that strength training can dramatically lower levels of blood fats, namely triglycerides and LDL cholesterol. This is powerfully positive news, since abnormal levels of blood fats are a risk factor for heart disease and should be checked periodically. LDL cholesterol is the harmful kind because it plugs up arteries. This condition eventually leads to atherosclerosis, which restricts and sometimes cuts off blood flow to vital organs.

Triglycerides are fats that travel in the blood and are eventually stored in fat cells. When too much of these fatty substances travels in the bloodstream, the excess gradually finds its way to the inner arterial walls, where it is deposited, eventually obstructing the arteries.

Develops Muscular Tone and Strength

Strength training develops your muscles by causing individual muscle fibers to enlarge. This gives your entire body the healthy look of firmness, otherwise known as muscle tone. Muscle tone basically means that your muscles are a little larger and more defined.

Strength training also builds strength, which technically means the amount of muscular force you can exert. You need strength for good health and an active life. Strong muscles protect and stabilize your joints and other connective tissues. They help you perform activities of daily living—carrying groceries, lifting children, mowing the lawn, toting luggage, and so forth—without stress and strain.

Strengthens Bones and Connective Tissue

Strength training not only builds muscle, it also builds bone by stimulating bone cells to produce more bone tissue. This effect has important implications in the prevention of osteoporosis, an age-related disease in which bones deteriorate. Although the exact mechanism hasn't been identified, connective tissues such as joints, ligaments, and tendons get stronger and denser too as a result of strength training.

IT'S TIME TO START CONTROLLING YOUR DIABETES

Now you have a better grasp of diabetes and what it takes to be in control of the disease. It's time to turn that knowledge into action with six steps that will help you manage your diabetes and shift it into reverse.

PART TWO

CONTROL DIABETES IN SIX EASY STEPS

STEP ONE

Follow a Healing, Healthy Diet

Imagine keeping your blood sugar at near-normal levels, requiring less medicine to control your blood sugar swings, or perhaps getting off diabetes drugs altogether, while avoiding the life-threatening complications of diabetes.

Is this possible? Absolutely—with a resolute commitment to a nutritious diet, coupled with an active lifestyle. And the earlier in the disease process you start making dietary changes, the greater the benefits.

But if you're like most people, with or without diabetes, altering dietary habits is like roller-skating up a hill. Too much trouble, so you go at it halfheartedly or don't even try. Sooner or later, another effort at dieting bites the dust.

So what's the solution? The best approach is to ease into healthier eating by making minor adjustments in your diet habits. Minor dietary adjustments can have a huge impact on your blood sugar control over time, as you will learn in this step. In addition, this step will:

- Cover six easy-to-follow nutrition principles to control your diabetes and transform the way you feel

- Provide a worksheet on which you can plan your meals
- Highlight three common meal-planning systems that are used in diabetes
- Discuss the pros and cons of using the glycemic index of foods
- Provide advice on how to simplify meal preparation
- Offer dietary tips on controlling your weight, cholesterol, triglycerides, and blood pressure

MINOR ADJUSTMENTS IN NUTRITION WORK BEST

Making full-scale changes in your diet all at once can be overwhelming, with a higher likelihood of failure. Begin with a few minor changes instead. You might start off by eating more fiber, then progress to trimming some fat from your diet. Here's an amazing fact: If you did just those two things, you'd start controlling your blood sugar almost automatically. By making small, gradual changes, you turn good diet intentions into second-nature habits, without much effort at all.

Once you get the hang of healthier eating, get a little more aggressive about your nutrition—with a plan that specifies the foods and nutrients you need each day. The plan doesn't have to be complicated, either, as you'll see. To get you started, here are six nothing-to-it nutrition principles to help you plan an effective diabetes-controlling diet.

Principle #1. Calculate Your Daily Calories

Before planning your meals, determine how many calories you need each day. Calories measure the amount of energy provided by food. The number of calories you need daily depends largely on your sex and level of activity:

- Generally, a woman who wants to maintain her weight can eat 1,800 to 2,000 calories a day (1,500 to 1,800 if she's sedentary).
- A woman who wants to lose weight can do so safely on a diet of 1,200 to 1,500 calories a day, particularly if she's moderately active.
- A man who wants to maintain his weight can eat 3,000 to 4,000 calories a day (1,800 to 2,000 if he's sedentary).
- A man who wants to lose weight can do so safely on a diet of 1,500 to 2,000 calories a day, particularly if he's moderately active.

Principle #2. Distribute Your Calories Among Carbohydrates, Protein, and Fat

According to current recommendations from the American Diabetes Association, 50 to 60 percent of the calories in your diet should come from carbohydrates, particularly fiber-rich complex carbohydrates, because they achieve better blood sugar control than simple carbohydrates do. In addition, strive to eat roughly the same amount of carbohydrates at each meal because this also helps stabilize your blood sugar levels.

Here's how to figure your carbohydrate needs based on a 2,000-calorie diet:

- Multiply calorie needs by 50 percent: $2{,}000 \times .50 = 1{,}000$ calories from carbohydrates.
- Divide 1,000 by 4, since there are 4 calories in a gram of carbohydrate: $1{,}000 \div 4 = 250$ grams of carbohydrate a day.
- Divide 250 grams by 5 (for breakfast, midmorning snack, lunch, midafternoon snack, and dinner): $250 \div 5 = 50$ grams of carbohydrate per meal or snack. (For the nutrient content

of various foods, it's a good idea to have a calorie and gram counter book or guide on hand.)

Regular servings of most carbohydrate foods contain about 15 grams of carbohydrate. For example:

1 small banana, peach, apple, or orange
½ grapefruit or pear
½ cup fruit juice
½ cantaloupe
2 tablespoons raisins
1 slice bread
¾ cup ready-to-eat cereal
½ cup cooked pasta
½ cup cooked beans
½ cup corn, peas, or yams
1 small (3-ounce) baked potato
½ bagel, English muffin, or bun
1 tortilla, waffle, or roll

Nonstarchy vegetables generally contain 5 grams of carbohydrate in each regular serving. For example:

½ cup cooked carrots, salad greens, green beans, brussels sprouts, broccoli, cauliflower, or spinach
1 cup raw carrots, radishes, or salad greens
1 large tomato

Protein intake should make up 10 to 20 percent of your total daily calories. (If you have kidney disease, you will be placed on a protein-restricted diet, since excess protein places an excess burden on the kidneys. Your doctor will recommend that you reduce your protein intake to around 10 percent of your daily calories—a smart strategy if you have diabetic-related kidney damage.)

As illustrated above with carbohydrates, here's how to figure your protein needs for a 2,000-calorie diet:

- Multiply your protein needs by 20 percent: $2{,}000 \times .20 = 400$ calories a day from protein.
- Divide 400 by 4, since there are 4 calories in a gram of protein: $400 \div 4 = 100$ grams of protein a day.
- Divide 100 grams by 3 for at least three meals that include protein (breakfast, lunch, and dinner, although it's wise to have an ounce or two of protein with snacks too): $100 \div 3 = 33$ grams of protein per meal or snack.

To help you plan: There are about 25 to 30 grams of protein in 4 ounces of white meat poultry, fish, and lean meat; 8 grams in a cup of skim milk or nonfat yogurt; and 18 grams in a 4-ounce serving of tofu. If you don't like to fuss with gram counting, just have a few ounces of protein with each meal, and you'll easily satisfy your protein requirement.

The balance of your calories should come from fat. If you eat the recommended amounts of carbohydrates and protein discussed above, this amount should add up to 30 percent or less of your total daily calories. Here's how you would figure your daily fat calories, particularly if you wanted to shoot for a lower intake of fat such as 20 percent (recommended):

- Multiply your fat requirement by 20 percent: $2{,}000 \times .20 = 400$ calories a day from fat.

- Divide 400 by 9, since there are 9 calories in a gram of fat: 400 ÷ 9 = 44 grams of fat a day.

Translating this into food, 44 grams of fat equates to:

½ cup of nuts
5 tablespoons of salad dressing
3 tablespoons of vegetable oil

For good health, most of your daily fat should come from polyunsaturated fats such as those found in vegetable oils, or monounsaturated fats like those found in olive oil or canola oil. The key is to follow a diet that is low in fat, particularly saturated fat, which brings us to the next principle.

Principle #3. Eat Less Fat

By slashing dietary fat (mainly saturated fat), you do your body a world of good. Reducing fat helps your body use insulin better, improves its use of glucose, cuts your risk of obesity, and protects against complications.

How, then, do you make the necessary cuts? Here are some tips:

- Use low-fat and skim-milk dairy products.
- Eat mostly fish, seafood, and skinless poultry, and small portions of lean cuts of beef.
- Use fats and oils sparingly in cooking and at the table.
- Use small amounts of salad dressings and spreads such as butter, margarine, and mayonnaise. Substitute low-fat or fat-free dressings on salads.

- Choose vegetable oils and soft margarines because they are lower in saturated fat than solid shortenings and animal fats. Remember, the healthiest fats you can select are the monounsaturated varieties, such as olive oil.
- Use as little fat as possible to cook vegetables and grains.
- Broil, bake, or microwave foods, rather than fry them.
- Season your foods with herbs, spices, lemon juice, and fat-free or low-fat salad dressings.
- Cut back on desserts, sweets, and candy, which are loaded with fat.
- Slash the fat from your diet by making healthful substitutions. For example, a baked potato for French fries, skim milk for whole milk, plain yogurt for sour cream or mayonnaise, ice milk or frozen yogurt for ice cream, a grilled chicken sandwich for a cheeseburger, fat-free pretzels for potato chips.

Principle #4. Eat a Variety of Foods

The greater the variety of foods you eat, the more health-building nutrients such as vitamins and minerals you get in your diet. That's significant because there's increasing evidence that these nutrients protect diabetics from serious complications, such as heart disease and kidney, eye, and nerve damage. A varied diet includes numerous servings of the following foods every day:

- Five or more servings of fresh fruits and vegetables. Examples of a serving: 1 medium piece of fruit, 1 cup of raw vegetables, ½ cup of cooked vegetables.
- Six or more servings of breads, whole grains, rice, and pasta (starches). Examples of a serving: ½ cup cooked whole-

grain cereal or rice, 2 rice cakes, 2 tacos, 1 medium baked potato or sweet potato.
- At least two servings of low-fat dairy products. Examples of a serving: 1 cup skim milk or yogurt, 1 cup nonfat cottage cheese, 2 ounces fat-free cheese.
- Two to three servings of protein-rich foods. Examples of a serving: 2 to 4 ounces of white meat chicken, fish, or lean red meat; ½ cup cooked beans or legumes; 1 egg. (Dairy products are also high in protein.)
- Fats and oils: Use these sparingly.

Principle #5. Eat More High-Fiber, Natural Foods

Eat foods as close as possible to the way they exist in nature: raw fruits; raw vegetables; frozen or lightly cooked vegetables; cooked beans and legumes; and natural, unrefined whole grains and cereals.

Why is this such a big deal? For one thing, these foods are packed with fiber, the nondigestible portion of plant foods. More fiber in your diet will help transform your eat-healthier efforts into something simple and automatic. You'll be able keep your blood sugar under better control, without constantly working at it or making yourself crazy.

The reason is that high-fiber foods break down into glucose more gradually and are absorbed more slowly into the bloodstream. They stabilize your blood sugar and do not cause postmeal surges. Shoot for a goal of 25 to 35 grams of fiber daily. (For a list of fiber-rich foods, refer to the box on page 90.)

In addition, if you have type 2 diabetes and take medicine, you may be able to eliminate or reduce your medication requirement by eating a diet high in natural carbohydrates and fiber. Case in point: In one study, 701 type 2 diabetics followed a high-fiber diet and exercised daily. Of these people, 207 were taking oral drugs to control their blood sugar levels, and 214 were using supplemental insulin. The rest were not on medication of any kind.

In just three weeks, 70 percent of those on oral medication were able to stop taking their medicine altogether; 36 percent of the insulin takers were able to discontinue the drug. Others in the study were able to reduce their medication requirement. There are two lessons here: Add more fiber to your diet, and stay active.

There's another reason for eating natural foods rather than processed ones: Natural foods are bursting with nutrients, each put to use in building and healing the body. Processed food, on the other hand, is nutritionally bankrupt and associated with various health problems.

Principle #6. Eat Multiple Meals

One of the best ways to keep your blood sugar level as close to normal as possible is to eat multiple meals throughout the day, preferably at the same time each day. Generally, this involves eating breakfast, lunch, and dinner, plus a midmorning snack and a midafternoon snack. Try to space your major meals four to five hours apart and leave at least two hours between meals and snacks to allow for adequate digestion.

At every meal, have a protein and a carbohydrate (preferably a natural, high-fiber carbohydrate). This combination of foods produces a slow release of glucose to keep your blood sugar stabilized and your energy level high throughout the day. What's more, your body works best when nutrients are replenished every few hours.

Here's an added benefit, particularly if you need to lose weight: Eating multiple meals can help you with weight control. Every time you eat a meal, your metabolic rate goes up. The reason is

FIBER RICH FOODS

FOOD	AMOUNT OF FIBER (IN GRAMS)
Figs, dried (10)	17
Ready-to-eat bran cereals (½ cup)	15
Wheat bran, raw (½ cup)	13
Prunes, dried (10)	8
Kidney beans, cooked (½ cup)	8
Navy beans, cooked (½ cup)	8
Black beans, cooked (½ cup)	7
Wheat germ, raw or toasted (½ cup)	7
Peas (½ cup)	7
Artichoke hearts (⅔ cup)	6
Dates, whole (10)	6
Potato (medium, baked with skin)	5
Pear (medium with skin)	5
Apricots, dried (10)	4
Barley (½ cup)	4
Garbanzo beans, cooked (½ cup)	4
Bulgur wheat, cooked (½ cup)	4
Whole kernel corn (½ cup)	3
Broccoli (½ cup)	3
Brussels sprouts (½ cup)	3
Squash, winter (½ cup)	3
Sweet potato (medium, baked, no skin)	3
Apple (medium, with skin)	3
Berries, any kind (½ cup)	3
Granola (½ cup)	3
Oatmeal, cooked (½ cup)	2
Brown rice, cooked (½ cup)	2

that your body starts working very hard to turn that meal into fuel. As part of digestion and absorption, heat is given off in a process called thermogenesis, and this elevates your metabolic rate. So by eating frequent meals throughout the day, your metabolism is constantly charged up, and your body burns calories more efficiently.

PRINCIPLES INTO PRACTICE

There you have it: six simple, practical changes that will serve up a menu for a healthier, more energetic life. The menu on page 92 shows you how these principles can be put into practice.

This menu is based on a requirement of 2,000 calories a day, with about 50 percent of those calories coming from carbohydrates, 20 percent from protein, and 25 percent from fat. In addition, this menu incorporates multiple meals—breakfast, lunch, dinner, and two snacks—and includes the suggested number of servings from various food groups. It is low in saturated fat, high in fiber from complex carbohydrates, and packed with vitamins and minerals.

On page 93 is a worksheet on which you can map out a similar menu. It makes meal planning a breeze.

Postscript: Along with your diet, be sure to drink eight to ten 8-ounce glasses of water daily, particularly since diabetes can cause dehydration. This occurs because the kidneys tend to use up lots of water to filter sugar from the blood.

OTHER MEAL-PLANNING TOOLS

Your doctor or dietitian may recommend a meal-planning system. These are nutrition tools that help you map out a day's or week's worth of menus. Three meal-planning systems are currently in vogue: *exchange lists, carbohydrate counting,* and the *diabetic food guide pyramid.* Here is a summary of how each one works.

Exchange Lists

One of the most enduring meal-planning systems for diabetes is the exchange list. Exchange lists are slates of similar foods grouped

MEAL	FOOD	SERVING SIZE	NUTRIENT GRAMS
Breakfast	Starch: Oatmeal	1 cup	25 g carb/6 g prot
	Starch: Mixed-grain toast	1 slice	12 g carb/3 g prot
	Protein: Poached egg	1	6 g prot/5 g fat
	Dairy: Skim milk	1 cup	12 g carb/8 g prot
	Fruit: Orange juice	¾ cup	21 g carb
	Fat: Canola soft margarine	1 tbsp	11 g fat
	Additional: _____	_____	_____
Midmorning Snack	Starch: Bran muffin	1	19 g carb/6 g fat
	Protein: _____	_____	_____
	Vegetable/Fruit: _____	_____	_____
	Dairy: Nonfat yogurt	1 cup	17 g carb/13 g prot
	Additional: _____	_____	_____
Lunch	Starch: Whole-wheat bread	2 slices	13 g carb/3g prot
	Vegetable: Tomato	1	6 g carb
	Protein: Turkey breast	2 ounces	16 g prot/9 g fat
	Dairy: _____	_____	_____
	Fruit: Banana	1	27 g carb
	Fat: Low-fat mayonnaise	1 tbsp	3 g carb/3 g fat
	Additional: Vegetable soup	1 cup	12 g carb
Midafternoon Snack	Starch: _____	_____	_____
	Protein: Low-fat Swiss cheese	1 ounce	1 g carb/8 g prot/1 g fat
	Vegetable/Fruit: Apple	1	32 g carb
	Dairy: _____	_____	_____
	Additional: _____	_____	_____
Dinner	Starch: Brown rice	1 cup	45 g carb/5 g prot
	Vegetable: Red beans	½ cup	20 g carb/6 g prot
	Vegetable: Green beans	1 cup	8 g carb/1 g prot
	Protein: Grilled salmon	4 ounces	31 g prot/13 g fat

Nutrition: Approximately 2,039 calories; 273 g carbohydrates (55% of calories from carbohydrates); 106 g protein (22% of calories from protein); and 48 g fat (22% of calories from fat). This menu also supplies 30 g of fiber.

MEAL	FOOD	SERVING SIZE	NUTRIENT GRAMS
Breakfast	Starch:		
	Starch:		
	Protein:		
	Dairy:		
	Fruit:		
	Fat:		
	Additional:		
Midmorning Snack	Starch:		
	Protein:		
	Vegetable/Fruit:		
	Dairy:		
	Additional:		
Lunch	Starch:		
	Vegetable:		
	Protein:		
	Dairy:		
	Fruit:		
	Fat:		
	Additional:		
Midafternoon Snack	Starch:		
	Protein:		
	Vegetable/Fruit:		
	Dairy:		
	Additional:		
Dinner	Starch:		
	Vegetable:		
	Vegetable:		
	Protein:		
	Fruit:		
	Fat:		
	Additional:		

together in categories (*exchanges*) with respect to their nutrient content. Each portion of food on the list has about the same amount of carbohydrate, protein, fat, and calories. Foods within the same group can be substituted for each other. For example, if your exchange allowance for protein at lunch was two proteins, you could choose one of the following: 2 ounces of smoked turkey, 2 ounces of chicken, or 1 ounce of cheese. Exchange lists give you the freedom and flexibility to exchange foods for each other as you plan your meals.

Specifically, foods on the exchange list are organized according to the following categories: starches, fruits, milk, other carbohydrates, vegetables, meat and meat substitutes, fat, combination foods (such as casseroles, pizza, pies, and so forth), and free foods.

Carbohydrate Counting

This is a method of counting the grams of carbohydrates you eat at meals and snacks. The reason for counting carbohydrates is that they have the most dramatic effect on your glucose levels. Your body converts carbohydrates into glucose faster than it does protein or fat. In fact, carbohydrates are converted to glucose within the first two hours after you eat a meal. So when you test your glucose two hours after eating, most of the surge in glucose comes from carbohydrates.

If you know how much carbohydrate you've eaten, you can predict what your blood glucose will do. A little bit of carbohydrate will elevate your glucose, and large amounts will make it go up even higher. For example, a full cup of cereal will make your blood glucose go higher than a half cup, and two cups will elevate it even more.

These metabolic facts of life have particular importance if you take insulin, which is required to balance the glucose. It is the amount of carbohydrate in a meal that largely determines how many units of insulin you require. Counting carbohydrates, therefore, can help you make appropriate insulin adjustments based on blood glucose patterns.

The Diabetes Food Guide Pyramid

Developed in 1995 by the American Diabetes Association and the American Dietetic Association, the diabetes food guide pyramid is a meal-planning system based on the 1994 United States Department of Agriculture's food guide pyramid. One of the tool's best features is that the pyramid illustration makes it easier to remember what to eat (see below). Practical and easy to use, the diabetes food guide pyramid places foods into six groups:

Grains, beans, and starchy vegetable group. This category

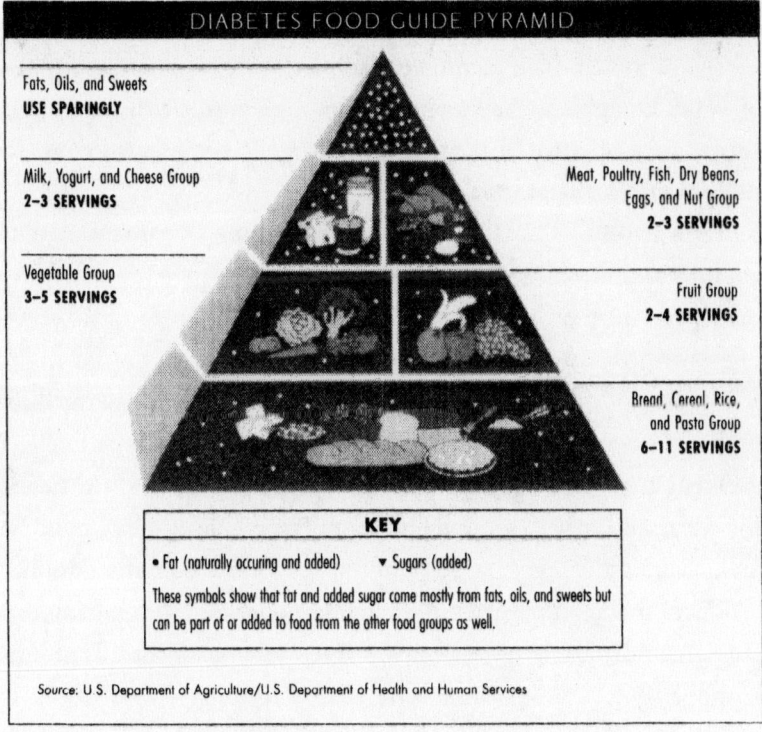

forms the broad base of the pyramid, implying that you should eat more foods from this group than any other. Each day, eat six or more servings from this group. Examples of a serving: 1 slice bread; ½ English muffin, bagel, or bun; 1 tortilla, waffle, or roll; ¾ cup ready-to-eat cereal; ½ cup cooked cereal; ½ cup cooked rice or pasta; ½ cup cooked beans; ½ cup corn, peas, or yams; 1 small (3-ounce) baked potato.

Vegetable group. Nonstarchy vegetables occupy the second tier of the pyramid. Each day, eat three to five servings of vegetables. Examples of a serving: ½ cup cooked carrots, salad greens, green beans, brussels sprouts, broccoli, cauliflower, or spinach; 1 cup raw carrots, radishes, or salad greens; ¼ cup vegetable juice.

Fruit group. Sharing the second tier of the pyramid with vegetables, fruits are generous contributors of carbohydrate, fiber, vitamins, and minerals to your diet. Each day, eat two to four servings of fruit. Examples of a serving: 1 small banana, peach, apple, or orange; ½ grapefruit or pear; ½ cantaloupe; ½ cup canned fruit (in its own juice); ¾ cup fruit juice.

Milk group. The third tier of the pyramid contains milk, yogurt, and cheese—foods that contribute carbohydrates, protein, and some fat to your diet. Each day, eat two to three servings from this group. Examples of a serving: 1 cup nonfat milk, ¾ cup nonfat plain yogurt, 1 cup nonfat or low-fat buttermilk, 1 ounce cheese.

Meat and others group. Also occupying the small third tier is the meat and others group. This category includes meat, poultry, fish, cheese, tofu, eggs, and peanut butter. Meats and other animal products are deemphasized in the pyramid because they are high in saturated fats. Each day, eat two to three servings from this group.

Examples of a serving: 2 to 3 ounces of white meat chicken, fish, or lean red meat; 1 egg; ½ cup cooked legumes.

Fats, sweets, and alcohol group. The tiny triangular tip of the pyramid contains foods that should be used sparingly in your diet. No recommended servings are provided from this group because they provide very few nutrients and are high in fat and calories.

USING A MEAL-PLANNING SYSTEM

No one meal-planning system or diet is perfect for every individual. The key is to find a system or diet that best fits you, your personal health needs, and your lifestyle. The box on pages 98–99 lists the advantages and disadvantages of each meal-planning system used in diabetes nutrition.

EATING OUT

When eating out, you can't measure portions as accurately as you can at home. Plus, portion sizes at restaurants are getting bigger in response to consumer demand. So chances are you're eating more than you think and probably packing away more calories. To help you gauge what's on your plate at a restaurant, use the following measurement equivalents:

- 2 ounces of cheese = one domino
- 1 serving of rice or cereal, or a potato = size of your fist
- 1 serving of vegetables or fruit = tennis ball
- 1 serving of meat, fish, or poultry = tape cassette, deck of cards, or palm of your hand

MEAL-PLANNING SYSTEMS

MEAL-PLANNING SYSTEM	FOOD GROUPS	HOW IT WORKS	ADVANTAGES	DISADVANTAGES
Exchange lists	Starches, fruits, milk, other carbohydrates, vegetables, meat and meat substitutes, fat, combination foods, and free foods	Substitute foods within the same group for each other	• Emphasizes a wide variety of foods • Is beneficial for weight control • Provides structure to make appropriate food choices	• Can be time consuming to plan
Carbohydrate counting	Same as exchange lists	The same amount of carbohydrates, counted in grams, is eaten at each meal to help control blood sugar	• Achieves better glucose control • Beneficial for people with type 1 diabetes who need to match insulin to the amount of carbohydrates eaten at meals	• Not as effective as other systems for weight loss • Requires regular monitoring of blood glucose levels before and after meals • Involves mathematical calculations

MEAL-PLANNING SYSTEMS (cont'd)

MEAL-PLANNING SYSTEM	FOOD GROUPS	HOW IT WORKS	ADVANTAGES	DISADVANTAGES
Diabetes food guide pyramid	Grain, beans, and starchy vegetable group; vegetable group; fruit group; milk group; meat and others group; fats, sweets, and alcohol group	Select the recommended number of daily servings from each of the six food groups	• Daily foods and servings spelled out • Nutrition principles in simple visual format • Weight control using lower number of servings from each food group • Plant-based foods useful for vegetarians • Adapts to ethnic foods • Works well for athletes, using higher number of servings and calories from each group	• Some people may choose too many high-calorie foods in each group, making weight control difficult • Not appropriate for diabetics who are visually impaired

THE GLYCEMIC INDEX: SAY SO LONG TO BLOOD SUGAR SWINGS

The glycemic index is a scale describing how fast a food is converted to glucose in your blood. Foods on the index are rated numerically, with glucose at 100. The higher the number assigned to a food, the faster it converts to glucose. Foods with a rating of 70 or higher are generally considered high-glycemic-index foods; a rating of 40 to 69, moderate-glycemic-index foods; and below 40, low-glycemic-index foods.

Foods with a high glycemic index are typically sugars and processed carbohydrates. But even some starchy carbohydrates have a high glycemic score, and fruits are scattered all over the index.

Scientists have measured responses to foods and have found that foods high on the scale tend to cause a rapid surge of insulin followed by a plunge of blood sugar that can lead to low energy. On the other hand, foods with a low glycemic index produce a slow, steady release of insulin and yield more sustained energy. Theoretically, you can use the index to select carbohydrates that are less likely to cause roller coaster swings in your blood sugar.

There are benefits to doing so. A number of studies have found that low-glycemic-index diets, on average, can reduce glycated hemoglobin, harmful cholesterol, and triglycerides. In addition, two well-designed studies, the Nurses' Health Study and the Health Professionals Follow-Up, demonstrated that eating large quantities of high-glycemic-index carbohydrates was linked to an increased risk of type 2 diabetes.

Even so, controversy simmers over the use of the index in diabetes. Here's why: Using the glycemic index to select foods can be misleading, for at least three reasons. First of all, meals do not consist of single foods. Normally, you eat mixed meals containing protein, carbohydrates, fiber, and some fat.

Mixed meals, thanks to their combination of protein, fiber, and fat, slow your digestion, providing a steady insulin release and therefore lowering the glycemic index of the entire meal. The point is, a food's rating on the index does not make much difference as long as it is eaten in slow-release food combinations.

The second problem with this method of rating foods is that some of the foods low on the index are simply not good for you, especially if you're trying to lose body fat. Ice cream, for example, is a low-glycemic-index food because it contains protein and fat, along with high-glycemic sucrose (sugar) and thus is broken down very slowly. Although it has a low glycemic index, it is chock-full of fat and sugar. Many foods with a low glycemic index can lead to unwanted body fat.

On the other hand, potatoes, cantaloupe, tropical fruits, and pumpkin have a relatively high glycemic index yet are loaded with vitamins, minerals, and fiber. Letting the glycemic index totally dictate what you eat is not always wise.

The third problem with using the glycemic index is that the ratings of foods can change, depending on their individual characteristics as well as how they are prepared. Take a banana. Its rating practically doubles with its ripeness! In addition, cooking starchy vegetables breaks down their cell walls, a process that increases their glycemic score.

Apart from diabetes management, the glycemic index has been used in sports nutrition and appetite research. Low-glycemic food eaten prior to long bouts of exercise have been found to extend endurance time. High-glycemic foods eaten after exercise are more effective at rapidly restoring muscle glycogen. In other research, low-glycemic foods have been deemed more filling than high-

GLYCEMIC INDEX OF CARBOHYDRATE FOODS (Glucose=100)

FOOD	GLYCEMIC INDEX	FOOD	GLYCEMIC INDEX
Bakery Products:		**Dairy Foods:**	
Waffles (Aunt Jemima)	76	Ice cream	36
Croissant	67	Chocolate milk	34
Bran muffin	60	Yogurt, low-fat, fruit	33
		Skim milk	32
Beverages:		Whole milk	27
Soft drink	68		
		Fruit and Fruit Products:	
Breads:		Raisins	64
Bagel	72	Orange juice	57
Bread, whole wheat	69	Banana	46
Taco shell	68	Grapes	43
Hamburger bun	61	Orange	43
Pita bread, white	57	Grapefruit	25
Breakfast Cereals:		**Legumes:**	
Corn flakes	84	Baked beans	48
Total cereal	76	Pinto beans	45
Shredded Wheat	69	Garbanzo beans	33
Grape-Nuts	67	Lima beans	32
Oatmeal, instant	65	Split peas, yellow	32
Oat bran	50	Black beans	30
All-Bran	42	Lentils	29
		Kidney beans	27
Cereal Grains:			
Cornmeal	69	**Pasta:**	
Rice, white	56	Instant noodles	47
Rice, brown	55	Macaroni	45
Bulgur	55	Spaghetti	41
		Ravioli, meat-filled	39
Cookies:			
Vanilla wafers	77	**Root Vegetables:**	
Graham crackers	74	Potato, baked	85
Oatmeal	54	Carrots	71
		Sweet potato	54
		Yam	51

GLYCEMIC INDEX OF CARBOHYDRATE FOODS* (cont'd)			
FOOD	GLYCEMIC INDEX	FOOD	GLYCEMIC INDEX
Snack Foods and Candies:		Sugars:	
Jelly beans	80	Honey	73
Corn chips	72	Fructose	23
Popcorn	55		
Chocolate bar	49	Vegetables:	
Peanuts	14	Corn	55
		Peas	48
Soups:			
Black bean	64		
Split pea	60		
Lentil	44		
Tomato	38		

*Index based on 50 grams of carbohydrate per serving.

Source: Foster-Powell K., and J. B. Miller. 1995. International tables of glycemic index. American Journal of Clinical Nutrition, 62 871S–90S.

glycemic foods. In the box above, you'll find the glycemic index of some common carbohydrate foods.

Even though it is important to understand the various effects foods have on insulin release, the glycemic index does not provide a complete picture. For healthy meal planning, diabetes experts recommend that you give priority to the amount of carbohydrate you eat, making sure that most of the carbohydrates in your diet are natural, rather than refined or processed. In addition, structure your meals to include a variety of foods. That way, you won't have to worry about the glycemic effect of foods you select.

SIMPLIFY MEAL PREPARATION

Don't let meal planning stress you out. There are ways to simplify the process so you can enjoy life:

- Cook in bulk. At the start of the week, cook large quantities of food ahead of time for the week ahead. This saves time and makes meal preparation a breeze. Refrigerate or freeze this food and reheat it when you need it.
- Chop up large quantities of salad vegetables and place them in a crisper. When you are ready for your next salad, it's right there in your refrigerator.
- Hard-boil eggs ahead of time and refrigerate them.
- Cook one-dish meals that contain multiple foods. Stews, soups, and casseroles are good examples. Prepare enough for two, four, or six meals. Then freeze the extras for future meals.
- For extra convenience, package soups, stews, or chili in single-serving portions. Freeze these foods in small, round, thin containers rather than in large, tall, rectangular containers so they will defrost more quickly.

FOOD RX FOR CONTROLLING DIABETES: CONQUER COMPLICATIONS

Controlling diabetes with diet becomes a little more challenging when certain health considerations come into play. Obesity, high cholesterol, high triglycerides, or hypertension call for intensified nutrition, with greater attention to calories, fat reduction, and food selections. With that in mind, here are several food prescriptions that will help you win back your good health from diabetes.

You Need to Lose Weight

People with type 1 or type 2 diabetes can be overweight, although the condition is more prevalent among those with type 2 diabetes. In fact, for people with type 2 diabetes, weight control is an integral part of medical therapy because it allows the body to better use insulin, thus lowering blood sugar.

Without question, it can be challenging to lose weight, especially if you're way off the ideal. But it's not impossible. What's more, you should have more motivation to get in shape than the average person. Losing weight substantially reduces your risk of life-threatening diabetic complications.

The first step is to eat fewer calories than your body uses each day. To lose one pound of body fat, you have to create a 3,500-calorie deficit, either by eating less, exercising more, or both. By cutting your total calorie intake by 500 calories each day, for example, you should be able to lose one pound a week (500 calories × 7 days)—a safe rate of weight loss. If you add exercise to this equation and burn any extra calories, your fat loss will be even greater. An hour of exercise, for example, can burn up anywhere from 250 to 500 calories.

Your weight-loss diet should be as low in fat as possible, since reducing dietary fat is one of the best ways to shed pounds. By keeping your total fat intake to 20 percent or less of total daily calories, you may be able to lose body fat with less restriction in total calories.

In addition, curb your intake of fat-forming foods such as sugar, processed foods, and alcohol. By curtailing these foods, along with fat, you'll automatically reduce the number of calories in your diet.

Losing weight can lower the total daily insulin you require, if you take insulin. In fact, your insulin needs will probably decrease with as little as a five-pound weight loss. Discuss insulin adjustments with your physician.

You Want to Keep Your Weight Off

Losing weight is the easy part. Keeping it off is harder. Most dieters regain as much as two-thirds of their lost pounds within a year and reacquire all of it within five years, according to the American Society of Bariatric Physicians.

First and foremost, staying trim requires a prudent, nutrient-rich diet. Match your calories to your activity level. The formula described earlier in this step can help you calculate the calories you require to maintain your weight. Also, keep your fat intake in the 20 to 25 percent range of your total daily calories by choosing low-fat foods.

Another maintenance tip: Eat plenty of high-fiber foods such as whole grains, fruits, vegetables, legumes, nuts, and seeds. A growing body of research shows that high-fiber eating helps peel off pounds and banish them for good.

How exactly does fiber work its weight-management magic? Mainly by curtailing your food intake. Because fibrous foods provide bulk, you feel full sooner, so you're less tempted to overeat. High-fiber foods also take longer to chew, so your meals last longer. That's a plus, since it takes about twenty minutes after starting a meal for your body to send signals to the brain that it's full.

Finally, get active and stay that way. Try to exercise most days of the week for at least thirty minutes each time. Discuss with your physician which type of exercise is a healthy choice for you. Regular exercise is one of the best ways to discourage the return of unwanted pounds.

Your Cholesterol Is Too High

With type 1 diabetes, you usually don't have to fret much about high cholesterol. People with type 1 diabetes tend to have normal, or better than normal, HDL counts. Nobody is sure why, but it may be due to supplemental insulin, which elevates HDL.

But it's another story altogether if you have type 2 diabetes. People with type 2 diabetes tend to be overweight, a condition that is associated with elevated LDL cholesterol and reduced HDL cholesterol.

If you have high levels of LDL cholesterol, you should reduce your total fat intake to 20 to 25 percent of your total calories and saturated fat to less than 7 percent. The remaining 10 to 15 percent should come from polyunsaturated and monounsaturated fats. Dietary cholesterol should be limited to less than 300 milligrams daily to discourage cardiovascular disease. Cholesterol is found in eggs, meats, and dairy products. Eating high-fiber foods, losing weight, and exercising will also bring your LDL cholesterol down.

Don't overindulge on sugary foods, either. Research has shown that sugar may be a risk factor for heart disease, possibly because it generates very-low-density lipoprotein cholesterol and triglycerides, both of which are harmful to the heart. Thus, avoid products listing more than 5 grams of sugar per serving on the label. If the specific amount of sugar is unlisted, stay away from products with sugar listed as one of the first four ingredients on the label. Sugar goes by various other names: sucrose, dextrose, maltose, lactose, maltodextrin, and corn syrup, to name just a few.

Your Triglycerides Are Too High

High triglycerides, which refer to fat circulating in the blood, are most often associated with type 2 diabetes and tend to occur simultaneously with high LDL and low HDL. Several factors can elevate your triglyceride levels: drinking alcohol, taking estrogen, and doing a poor job controlling your diabetes. Higher-carbohydrate diets tend to increase triglycerides too. So does eating too much high-fructose corn syrup, a refined version of fructose made from corn and found in many processed foods and beverages.

If your diabetes is complicated by high triglycerides (over 250 mg/dl), the American Diabetes Association suggests that you try a higher-fat diet with 40 percent of your total daily calories derived from fat. However, half your fat should come from monounsaturated fats, which have been shown in research to lower triglyceride levels. A higher monounsaturated fat diet might include olive oil, canola oil, peanut oil, or sesame oil as fat servings, or servings of nuts and seeds as part of your daily diet. When you increase your calories from fat, be careful not to increase your total calories, particularly if you're trying to watch your weight.

You Have High Blood Pressure

A diet designed to control blood glucose is also beneficial for reducing high blood pressure (hypertension). That's because these diets are rich in nutrients such as calcium, potassium, and magnesium, all of which help normalize blood pressure.

One mineral that should be restricted, however, is sodium, found in table salt. Too much salt in the body tends to narrow the diameter of blood vessels. Then the heart has to work harder to pump the same amount of blood, and blood pressure goes up as a result. Excessive salt also makes the body retain too much water, and this may cause a rise in blood pressure.

If you suffer from high blood pressure, do not add salt to your food, and avoid salty foods such as chips, smoked meats, pickled foods, cheese and cheese products, fast foods, and canned foods. If you miss the taste of salt on foods, try a salt substitute or experiment with various herbs and spices when cooking.

Losing weight reduces blood pressure too. On average, you can cut your blood pressure by several points by losing weight through diet and exercise.

Another way to reduce high blood pressure is with aerobic exercise, such as walking, jogging, running, swimming, bicycling, and so forth. Most studies of hypertensive people show that a reduction can occur with as little as three exercise sessions a week for thirty to sixty minutes each time.

• • •

WHAT THE EXPERTS ADVISE
Top-Ten Strategies for Eating a Healthy, Healing Diet
Lori Bender, M.S., R.D., C.D.E.

Lori Bender is a certified diabetes educator and a nutrition consultant for long-term care facilities, hospitals, industry, and private clients. She has written *Something's Cooking*, which not only contains original recipes from various ethnic groups but also recommends changes that can be made to alter the recipes for specific diets. She developed a newsletter for a disease management company called *Diabetes Solutions* and has written articles for the *Consulting Nutritionists' Newsletter* and *Florida Woman*. Here are her top-ten strategies for controlling diabetes with a healing, healthy diet.

1. Make healthy food choices. A well-nourished body gets sick less often, and people with diabetes are at risk for numerous complications. Choose foods from all the food groups (breads and starches, meats, vegetables, fruit, dairy, and fat); foods that are colorful and not overcooked, because they contain more vitamins and minerals; foods that are fresh rather than processed (which tend to be higher in sugar, salt, and preservatives); and foods that are lower in fat

content. Also choose a variety; don't stick to just a few limited foods.

2. Eat less saturated fat, the type of fat that is solid at room temperature. Many meat and animal products are high in saturated fat, including hamburger meat, cheese, bacon, and butter. Eat very lean beef once or twice a week because beef is high in iron.

3. Choose fish and poultry more often than red meat because they are lower in calories. Fish also contains polyunsaturated fat and omega-3 fatty acids. Be sure to remove the skin from poultry because it is full of saturated fat and cholesterol.

4. Eat foods that are high in fiber: fruits, vegetables, whole grains, and beans. When eating fruits and vegetables, eat the skins (if they are edible) because they are high in fiber.

5. Eat about the same amount of food daily and keep your meal times consistent. This will help keep your blood sugar more stable.

6. Do not skip meals—your blood sugar may drop too low.

7. Try not to eat meals or snacks too close together. Wait about three hours between any meal and snack to allow time for digestion.

8. Include a protein food with every meal and snack. Protein takes longer than bread or starches to turn to blood sugar. Protein is found in meats, poultry, fish, cheese, and eggs.

9. There are no longer any special or restricted foods in diabetes nutrition. The same food you prepare for your family is what you can eat too. The only difference is that you need to watch your portions and be careful to not have too many carbohydrates (breads and starches) at any one meal or snack.

10. Sucrose (simple sugar) is not bad anymore. One portion of a food containing sugar, such as a piece of cake, will increase your blood sugar the same amount as one portion of a food containing complex carbohydrates, such as a slice of whole-wheat bread. The difference is that simple sugar acts faster than complex carbohydrates do, so you should not eat simple sugar too often.

STEP TWO

Drive Diabetes into Retreat with Natural Remedies

Step 2 is like a sequel to Step 1—the next episode of nutrition where you learn about using dietary supplements to control your diabetes. In this step, you'll find out about the major supplemental nutrients involved in the treatment of diabetes and the prevention of its complications, including:

- Antioxidants
- B vitamins
- Antidiabetic minerals
- Amino acids
- Supplemental fats
- Herbs

You'll also learn about how these supplements work to fight diabetes and what dosage to take for a beneficial effect. There's a lot here, but it's a lot that can help you. Always get your physician's okay before taking dietary supplements.

SUPERSTAR ANTIOXIDANTS

One surefire way to better control your diabetes is to get enough antioxidants. Supplied by food and supplements and produced internally by your own body, antioxidants are nutrients with the power to disarm disease-causing free radicals.

Among the antioxidants important to people with diabetes are beta-carotene and other carotenoids, vitamin C, vitamin E, and specialized antioxidants such as alpha-lipoic acid and coenzyme Q10 (CoQ10). They work in near-miraculous ways to arrest free radicals. It's hard to say enough about the protective power of these vital nutrients!

But here's the rub: Scientists have discovered that people with diabetes have low levels of antioxidants in their bodies, a condition that leads to oxidative stress. This develops when free radicals start outnumbering antioxidants. Oxidative stress further depletes antioxidants, injures tissues, and leaves you vulnerable to diseases.

Oxidative stress is markedly elevated in type 1 and type 2 diabetes. One of the major causes of oxidative stress is elevated glucose (hyperglycemia), which enfeebles your body's own force of internally produced antioxidants. When antioxidant defenses are weakened, you're left vulnerable to a range of free-radical-generated diseases. Topping the list are heart disease and other diabetic complications such as nephropathy and retinopathy.

Make no mistake about it: To better control your diabetes, you must shore up your antioxidant defenses, and you can do this by consuming antioxidants from food and from dietary supplements. The information that follows explains specific antioxidants that are particularly helpful in controlling both type 1 and type 2 diabetes.

BETA-CAROTENE AND THE CAROTENOIDS

The most colorful foods—apricots, mangoes, strawberries, carrots, sweet potatoes, red bell peppers, tomatoes, broccoli, and so forth—are brimming with plant pigments called *carotenoids*. These nutrients help ward off many diseases and are useful in preventing diabetic complications.

The first carotenoid to be isolated was beta-carotene, which gives carrots and other vegetables their characteristic orange color. In your body, beta-carotene is converted to vitamin A on an as-needed basis. As an antioxidant, beta-carotene's main role is to detoxify free radicals. This amazing nutrient can also destroy free radicals after they're formed.

Today, scientists have discovered more than six hundred carotenoids in nature and are reporting that many may be a hundred times more powerful than beta-carotene and other antioxidants alone. The main carotenoids now under investigation are alpha-carotene, cryptoxanthin, gamma-carotene, lutein, and lycopene—all found mostly in fruits and vegetables.

How Carotenoids Help Control Diabetes

To date, the research into carotenoids and diabetes has focused mainly on deficiency issues. Evidence has cropped up that people with diabetes (type 1 and type 2) have dangerously low levels of these protective nutrients in their bodies. With carotenoids in short supply, you could be at greater risk for diabetic complications. Thus, increasing your fruit and vegetable consumption, plus taking supplemental carotenoids such as beta-carotene, may be therapeutic.

VITAMIN C

Also known as ascorbic acid, vitamin C is a water-soluble nutrient that can be synthesized by many animals but not by humans. It is an essential nutrient in our diets and functions primarily in the formation of connective tissues such as collagen. Vitamin C is also involved in immunity, cholesterol reduction, and wound healing. As an antioxidant, vitamin C keeps free radicals from destroying the outermost layers of cells.

This nutrient is found mostly in citrus fruits, cantaloupe, strawberries, green and red peppers, and numerous green vegetables.

How Vitamin C Helps Control Diabetes

As a diabetic, you require more vitamin C. Here's why: Insulin helps ferry vitamin C into cells, but excessive levels of blood glucose inhibit this process. Consequently, diabetics may have concentrations of vitamin C in their cells that are 30 percent lower than in people without diabetes. If this deficiency becomes chronic and goes uncorrected, you're susceptible to conditions that can aggravate your health. Specifically, here's how vitamin C can help.

Reduces glycation. Long-term complications of diabetes such as heart, kidney, eye, and nerve diseases can be caused by glycation, in which glucose links up (or glycates) with hemoglobin, a component of red blood cells that carries oxygen in the blood from the lungs to the tissues, and albumin, the most highly concentrated protein in blood. Glucose can also bind to other substances in the body, including red blood cells and white blood cells. A by-product of glycation is the production of advanced glycated end products (AGEs), which can inflict damage in your body.

Whenever such a linkage occurs, cells, proteins, and other substances no longer work normally because their structure and function have been modified. And that's bad news. For example, modified hemoglobin clings to oxygen instead of releasing it normally. Consequently, cells become starved for oxygen.

Other problems arise as well. Glycated red blood cells have a shortened life span. Glycated white blood cells are unable to fight infection. Molecules of LDL cholesterol can become glycated too, a process that prevents the normal shutdown of cholesterol synthesis in the liver. As a result, cholesterol levels soar, increasing the risk of atherosclerosis. Also, AGEs (the glycated substances) generate health-damaging free radicals.

The bottom line: When blood glucose is chronically elevated, there is a glut of glycated cells and substances in your system. Your body can't handle the excess, and the risk of complications increases.

Vitamin C to the rescue. Studies show that vitamin C significantly reduces glycation, particularly of proteins, although scientists are unclear why. Based on current research, 500 to 3,000 milligrams daily of vitamin C appears to counteract the formation of glycated proteins.

Inhibits the buildup of sorbitol. Under normal circumstances, glucose is metabolized, or broken down, to form carbon dioxide and water in the production of energy. When there is too much glucose in your bloodstream, the excess is metabolized into a product called sorbitol. Unfortunately, sorbitol tends to build up in the body, damaging and even destroying cells and tissues. This accumulation plays a huge role in the development of long-term complications of diabetes.

Vitamin C can significantly reduce sorbitol levels, at dosages ranging from 250 to 1,000 milligrams daily, according to research. In one study involving type 1 diabetics, supplementation with vitamin C normalized sorbitol levels within thirty days.

VITAMIN E

Vitamin E is a fat-soluble vitamin, meaning that it can be stored with fat in the liver and other tissues. Vitamin E is also a component of cells, sandwiched between the fatty layers that make up cell membranes. When free radicals come along, they hitch up to vitamin E, damaging it instead of the rest of the cell membrane. In the process, vitamin E soaks up the free radicals, and the cell is protected from harm. Vitamin C and other antioxidants can regenerate vitamin E. But with a shortage of vitamin E, there is an increase in free radicals, cellular injuries, and subsequent disorders to bodily tissues.

Vitamin E is thus an important antioxidant that protects cells from damage. Specifically, vitamin E prevents a free-radical-initiated process known as lipid peroxidation. In a domino-like series of chemical reactions, free radicals hook up with fatty acids in the body to form substances called peroxides. Peroxides attack cell membranes, setting off a chain reaction that creates many more free radicals.

In addition, vitamin E protects beta-carotene from destruction in the body and is an important guardian of blood vessel health. Vitamin E also interrupts the plaque-forming process that can clog your arteries.

Foods high in vitamin E include vegetable oils, nuts, and seeds.

How Vitamin E Helps Control Diabetes

Vitamin E is a powerful antioxidant that helps reduce the complications of diabetes by improving insulin action and combating oxidative stress.

Regulates blood sugar. In a study of vitamin E's effect on glucose metabolism and insulin action, ten control (healthy) subjects and fifteen people with type 2 diabetes underwent an oral glucose tolerance test before and after taking 900 milligrams of vitamin E daily for four months. In the control group, vitamin E improved the action of insulin and the body's handling of glucose. In the diabetic patients, these benefits were even more pronounced, suggesting that vitamin E is a useful nutrient for blood sugar control.

Reduces glycation. As explained above, glycation is the binding of glucose to proteins or to other substances. Research indicates that supplemental vitamin E at just 100 IU daily significantly lowers glycated hemoglobin. Thus, vitamin E may be useful in preventing long-term complications of diabetes.

May help prevent retinal and kidney problems. Among the most-feared long-term consequences of diabetes are kidney damage (nephropathy) and retinal disease (retinopathy). Based on the results of a preliminary study, vitamin E supplementation may normalize markers for these conditions.

A marker is a physiological signpost, usually pinpointed in blood or urine tests, that a certain disease or condition may be on the horizon. A marker for retinopathy is reduced blood flow to the retina, and a marker for nephropathy is abnormal levels of creatinine in the blood. Used to evaluate kidney function, creatinine is a breakdown product of creatine, an energy-producing constituent of muscle. The kidneys excrete creatinine. When your kidneys are functioning normally, concentrations of creatinine in the blood remain constant and normal.

The study in question included fifty patients with type 1 diabetes and thirteen people without the disease. The subjects took either 1,300 IU of vitamin E a day, or a placebo, for four months. Although the diabetic patients had no retinopathy or nephropathy, their retinal blood flow was reduced, and their creatinine levels were abnormally elevated—markers indicating that diabetic complications could occur.

Four months of vitamin E treatment, however, normalized these markers. Retinal blood flow returned to normal, as did creatinine levels. This study hints at vitamin E's ability to prevent retinopathy and nephropathy, but the researchers noted that additional research, with larger numbers of subjects, is needed to substantiate these findings.

Fights heart and blood vessel disease. Heart disease is responsible for more than 70 percent of deaths in diabetes. In fact, heart disease and stroke are two to four times more common in people with diabetes. Vitamin E, however, may prove to be a mighty sentry against these deadly complications.

In a fourteen-week study of twenty-one patients, researchers at the University of Texas Southwestern Medical Center found that taking 1,200 IU of vitamin E daily reduced LDL cholesterol oxidation—a process that, if not stopped, can lead to clogged arteries.

SPECIALIZED ANTIOXIDANTS: ALPHA-LIPOIC ACID

Alpha-lipoic acid is a highly researched antioxidant that has several vital duties in the body. Like a traffic cop at the cellular level, this nutrient directs calories from fats and carbohydrates into energy production. More specifically, it is involved in breaking down fats and carbohydrates into fatty acids and blood sugar so they can be converted into fuel for energy. Thus, alpha-lipoic acid is a key factor in metabolism.

As an antioxidant, alpha-lipoic acid also protects the body against disease and works with other antioxidants such as vitamin

C, vitamin E, and beta-carotene to destroy free radicals. In the process, antioxidants are often temporarily wounded. However, they can be regenerated back to their original form by other antioxidants. Alpha-lipoic acid is an antioxidant with the power to do this.

In addition, alpha-lipoic acid is a destroyer itself. It extinguishes a free radical known as the hydroxyl radical, which is highly damaging to the body.

Alpha-lipoic acid also helps produce glutathione in cells. Glutathione is an important internally produced antioxidant that regenerates immune cells, prevents cholesterol from becoming toxic, and deactivates cancer-causing substances.

Alpha-lipoic acid is often referred to as the "universal antioxidant." Here's why: It is fat-soluble, which means it can work its protective powers within the lipid-rich membranes of cells. It is also water-soluble, which means it can work within the cell's interior. In other words, alpha-lipoic acid exerts a dual defense. If free radicals infiltrate the cell walls, they are apprehended inside the cells. There's no getting past alpha-lipoic acid.

This antioxidant is manufactured by the body, but found in small amounts in potatoes, yams, spinach, and red meats.

How Alpha-Lipoic Acid Helps Control Diabetes

Used therapeutically in Germany for more than thirty years as an approved drug to treat diabetic complications, alpha-lipoic acid is a potent weapon against the disease for a number of reasons. Here are the details.

Repairs nerve damage. A long-term complication of diabetes is nerve damage (neuropathy), which is caused by high blood sugar and, quite possibly, by a lack of antioxidants in nerve cells. Symptoms are pain, tingling, and numbness in the hands and feet.

Research with alpha-lipoic acid shows that it increases blood flow to nerves, eases symptoms, repairs nerve damage, and stimulates the regeneration of nerve fibers.

In one study, seventy-three patients with type 2 diabetes were given either 800 milligrams of alpha-lipoic acid, or a placebo, daily for four months. By the end of the experimental period, the placebo takers continued to experience nerve deterioration, but in those who took alpha-lipoic acid, there was nerve regeneration.

Alpha-lipoic acid may ease the symptoms of nerve damage too. In one study, 328 diabetics with nerve damage took 600 milligrams a day of alpha-lipoic acid, or a placebo, daily for three weeks. By the end of the study, the alpha-lipoic-acid supplementers had fewer symptoms than those who took the placebo.

Lowers blood sugar levels. By promoting glucose metabolism, alpha-lipoic acid effectively lowers blood sugar levels, according to research. In one study, lean and obese individuals with type 2 diabetes were given 600 milligrams of alpha-lipoic acid twice a day for four weeks. Supplementation improved blood sugar metabolism and made body cells more responsive to insulin.

Reduces glycation. Like vitamin C and vitamin E, alpha-lipoic acid reduces glycation, the process by which glucose attaches to proteins in the body, creating abnormal proteins called AGEs. Over time, AGEs damage the body and lead to long-term complications of diabetes. Taking alpha-lipoic acid can help prevent such complications by interfering with the formation of AGEs.

SPECIALIZED ANTIOXIDANTS: COENZYME Q10

As an antioxidant, coenzyme Q10 (abbreviated as CoQ10) protects cell membranes from free-radical assaults. This substance is also found naturally inside the mitochondria—the energy factories of cells—where it is involved in the conversion of food to energy.

CoQ10 is highly concentrated in your heart muscle cells, which require vast amounts of energy to keep the heart pumping its volumes of blood—about 75 gallons every hour. Supplementally, this nutrient appears to have many heart-healthy properties. For example, it helps keep arteries clog free, lowers blood pressure, and improves cardiac efficiency. CoQ10 also strengthens the immune system and may enhance the quality of overall health. Many studies have been done supporting CoQ10's benefits as an oral supplement.

CoQ10 is made by the body, but is also available from seafood.

How Coenzyme Q10 Helps Control Diabetes

Scientists are only beginning to scratch the surface of CoQ10's potential benefits to people with diabetes, but the findings are promising. One thing is certain, though: Research has found that diabetics have low levels of this antioxidant in their bodies, a deficiency that may hustle patients toward serious diabetic complications. Here's how CoQ10 can help.

May improve beta cell function. Studies in Japan, where most of the research has been conducted on CoQ10 and diabetes, suggest that the supplement may improve the function of insulin-producing beta cells in cases of type 2 diabetes in which beta cell function may be impaired.

May treat cardiac complications. Because of its benefits in treating heart disease, CoQ10 has been investigated as a supplemental therapy for people with diabetes who have cardiac complications. According to medical literature on CoQ10 and diabetes, the supplement has been shown to reduce irregular heartbeats in cardiac patients, including those with diabetes. In heart patients, CoQ10 (60 milligrams twice daily) also decreased blood pressure and improved insulin resistance. It may also be helpful in treating cardiomyopathy, a potentially life-threatening weakening of the heart muscle that often plagues people with diabetic-related heart disease.

THE B COMPLEX VITAMINS: OTHER GOOD-FOR-YOU NUTRIENTS

In addition to the nutrients described above, make sure your diet supplies ample amounts of B complex vitamins. Vital for energy, B complex vitamins are involved in nearly every reaction in the body, from the manufacture of new red blood cells to the metabolism of carbohydrates, fats, and protein.

How B Complex Vitamins May Help Control Diabetes

Found in a wide variety of plant and animal foods, this important family of nutrients has several members that appear to enhance the body's use of insulin and improve the metabolism of glucose.

Biotin is involved in metabolism, helping your body make and use fats and amino acids. It steps up the activity of an enzyme called glucokinase, which is responsible for helping the liver utilize glucose. In diabetes, glucokinase concentrations are in short supply. According to research, high-dose biotin supplementation (16 milligrams daily) improves glucokinase activity and glucose metabolism in people with type 1 diabetes.

Vitamin B_1 (thiamine) plays a key role in the production of energy. In addition, it is essential for the maintenance of a good appetite, normal digestion, and the health of the gastrointestinal tract. In diabetes, there can be a deficiency of this vitamin, possibly warranting supplementation.

Vitamin B_3 (niacin) is involved in the metabolism of carbohydrates, fats, and protein and is essential for the health of the nervous system, skin, and digestive system. Some compelling evidence points to a therapeutic benefit of taking niacin in the form of supplemental niacinamide if you have recent-onset type 1 diabetes. It appears to help restore beta cells and prevent type 1 diabetes from progressing. The dosages used in studies were calculated according to body weight: 25 milligrams per kilogram (2.2 pounds) of body weight.

Vitamin B_6 (pyroxidine) influences nearly every system in the body. For example, it assists in creating amino acids, turning carbohydrates into glucose, metabolizing fats, producing neurotransmitters (chemicals that relay nerve impulses), and manufacturing antibodies to ward off infection.

Also, vitamin B_6 prevents the buildup of homocysteine in the blood, a toxic by-product of the amino acid methionine that can eventually lead to atherosclerosis (hardening of the arteries).

Supplemental vitamin B_6 appears to guard against the development of diabetic neuropathy, as well as other complications of diabetes, probably because it blocks the glycation of proteins. Vitamin B_6 might be of some value in treating gestational diabetes too. In one study, taking 100 milligrams of the nutrient daily for only two weeks eliminated the gestational diabetes disease in twelve out of fourteen women.

Vitamin B_{12} (cobalamin) regulates many functions in the body. Among the most vital is the production of red blood cells. Vitamin B_{12} is the director in this process, making sure that enough cells are manufactured. Without vitamin B_{12} red blood cell production falls off, and the result is misshapen cells and anemia.

Intravenously or orally, vitamin B_{12} supplementation has been used to treat diabetic neuropathy. One reason is that vitamin B_{12} is important to the health of your nervous system.

Pantothenic acid is a B complex vitamin that plays in many roles in your body. The name *pantothenic acid* comes from the Greek word *pantothen*, which means "everywhere"—an apt derivative, since this nutrient is present in every living cell. First recognized as a substance that stimulates growth, pantothenic acid is quite active in metabolism. Additionally, pantothenic acid is involved in immunity, wound healing, the formation of hormones, and the regulation of nerve impulses.

In the treatment of diabetes, pantothenic acid in the form of pantethine has been used to lower blood lipids in patients undergoing dialysis and to improve platelet function.

Inositol is involved primarily in normal fat metabolism. It helps prevent dangerous buildups of fat in the arteries and keeps the liver, heart, and kidneys healthy. This nutrient is also required by cells in the bone marrow, eye membranes, and intestines for proper growth. In diabetes, it has been used to treat diabetic neuropathy, usually in the range of 1,000 to 2,000 milligrams a day.

ANTIDIABETIC MINERALS

Minerals are vital for the formation of body structures such as bones and tissue and are involved in many physiological processes, including metabolism and energy production. Several minerals are important in diabetes management and may be useful in preventing or slowing diabetic complications.

CALCIUM

Of all minerals in your body, calcium is the most abundant. It accounts for 40 percent of your skeleton, and about 99 percent of the calcium in your body is deposited in bones and teeth. These structures are hardened and strengthened by calcium, working in combination with the mineral phosphorus. The remaining percent of the body's calcium is concentrated in the soft tissues where it plays an essential role in muscle contraction, nerve transmission, blood coagulation, and the activity of the heart.

Foods rich in calcium include dairy products, kale, turnip greens, and broccoli.

How Calcium May Help Control Diabetes

Although calcium is vital for bone health, it is being studied for other health benefits. For example, emerging research hints that it may promote normal insulin action. In one study, researchers gave 1,500 milligrams of calcium, or a placebo, to twenty nondiabetic patients for eight weeks. Supplementation decreased fasting glucose levels and promoted insulin sensitivity. Even though this trial did not test people with diabetes, the findings suggest the usefulness of calcium in controlling diabetes.

Calcium supplementation also appears to counteract a side effect that can occur while taking the oral diabetes drug metformin (Glucophage). Up to 30 percent of people who are prescribed metformin show signs of reduced absorption of vitamin B_{12}, a nutrient that relies on calcium for uptake by cells. A study conducted at the Mount Sinai School of Medicine in New York City found that oral supplementation with calcium cleared up the B_{12} absorption problems associated with this drug.

For more than twenty years, scientists have known that ample calcium helps control and prevent high blood pressure. This should be compelling information if you have diabetes, because high blood pressure is often a complication of the disease.

CHROMIUM

If ever there was a "diabetes mineral," chromium may be it. That's because chromium's main assignment in the body is to help turn carbohydrates into glucose. Chromium also helps regulate and produce the hormone insulin. In fact, chromium makes insulin work more efficiently in the body, and without it, insulin simply would not function.

Good sources of chromium include brewer's yeast, nuts, cheese, whole grains, oysters, and mushrooms.

How Chromium May Help Control Diabetes

Decades of research show that chromium supplementation lessens and even reverses the symptoms of diabetes, particularly type 2. The reasons for this are clear: Chromium helps insulin regulate and normalize blood sugar, as well as decrease requirements for insulin and oral diabetes medications. It also improves your body's ability to transport blood glucose into cells.

Other research indicates that chromium supplementation:

- Improves glucose tolerance and can restore it to normal
- Enhances insulin secretion
- Reduces fasting glucose and insulin levels in gestational diabetes
- Decreases triglycerides

- Promotes more favorable cholesterol levels
- Encourages the loss of body fat
- Promotes muscular gains

MAGNESIUM

Magnesium is the maestro of more than four hundred metabolic reactions in your body. It helps orchestrate the protein-making machinery inside the cells of soft tissues; it helps direct the metabolism of potassium, calcium, and vitamin D; it is necessary for the release of energy; it helps your muscles relax after contracting; it is involved in glucose metabolism; and it plays a central role in the secretion and action of insulin.

Diabetes experts have known for some time that people with type 1 and type 2 diabetes are often deficient in magnesium. This deficiency is most likely related to increased losses of urinary magnesium as a result of chronic glycosuria (glucose in the urine).

In people with type 2 diabetes, magnesium deficiency makes the body's cells less sensitive to insulin, according to a number of studies. Severe magnesium deficiency can cause abnormalities in the function of the heart and is possibly related to cardiovascular disease, heart attack, and high blood pressure.

How do you know if you're magnesium needy? There's no truly accurate way to measure or detect a magnesium deficiency, and the American Diabetes Association doesn't recommend routine testing of magnesium status if you're otherwise healthy but have diabetes.

Foods high in magnesium include garbanzo beans, beet greens, fruits, and whole grains.

How Magnesium May Help Control Diabetes

Bodily stores of magnesium are valuable in helping the body handle glucose and maintain proper blood levels. So say several studies, including one in which magnesium supplementation (400 milligrams daily) given to nonobese elderly subjects showed significant improvements in insulin action and glucose tolerance.

Even so, the case for magnesium therapy isn't yet proved. The American Diabetic Association feels that more clinical trials are needed to demonstrate convincingly that magnesium supplementation will cut the incidence of diabetes and its complications.

POTASSIUM

Potassium serves the body in many ways. It assists the nerves in sending messages, helps digestive enzymes do their work, ensures proper muscle functioning (including that of the heart), regulates water balance, and releases energy from protein, carbohydrates, and fats. A potassium deficiency can lead to irregular heartbeats, high blood pressure, muscular weakness, fatigue, kidney and lung problems, and insulin resistance.

Bananas, potatoes, lima beans, flounder, and winter squash are all high in potassium.

How Potassium May Help Control Diabetes

Because of potassium's close connection to insulin resistance, it is important to guard against a deficiency by eating a balanced diet, rather than by taking supplements. A case, however, might be made for potassium supplements as a treatment for high blood pressure, a frequent complication of diabetes. Research indicates that daily dosages ranging from 2.5 to 5 grams of supplemental potassium can significantly reduce blood pressure in hypertensive patients. But talk to your doctor before pursuing this avenue of therapy.

VANADIUM

Named after the Scandinavian goddess of beauty and youth, vanadium is a building material of bones and teeth. It is also associated with proper glucose regulation. Vanadium acts like insulin in the body and has been shown to enhance its effects, which is why this trace mineral has been intensely researched for its role in the management of diabetes. The supplemental form of vanadium is vanadyl sulfate. Food sources of vanadium include skim milk, lobster, vegetables, vegetable oils, butter, and cheese.

How Vanadium May Help Control Diabetes

Although nutritional researchers have studied vanadium for more than forty years, the mineral is not yet considered essential for humans (it is essential for plants and animals). Many scientists, however, have been rethinking this position. In 1994, an article published in the *Journal of the American Dietetic Association* presented evidence that vanadium may indeed be an essential nutrient in our diets.

The attention paid to vanadium has to do mostly with diabetes. Research indicates that vanadium may:

- Improve fasting glucose levels and insulin resistance in type 2 diabetes (50 milligrams twice daily of vanadyl sulfate)
- Enhance insulin sensitivity in type 2 diabetes (100 milligrams daily of vanadyl sulfate)
- Lower the insulin requirement in type 1 diabetes (125 milligrams daily)

ZINC

Zinc is at the heart of many activities in your body. For example, it helps absorb vitamins; break down carbohydrates; synthesize nucleic acid, which directs the manufacture of protein in cells; and regulate the growth and development of reproductive organs. Zinc is also a component of insulin, and it prevents deficiencies that can lead to problems in your body's use of insulin.

A moderate zinc deficiency can occur in people with type 1 and type 2 diabetes, although it is not clear why. Zinc-poor diets are also associated with cardiovascular disease, high blood pressure, elevated triglycerides, and impaired glucose tolerance.

Meat, poultry, shellfish, and whole grains are all well endowed with zinc.

How Zinc May Help Control Diabetes

Very few studies have been conducted regarding zinc supplementation for people with diabetes. In one study, however, twenty-two patients with type 1 diabetes received 30 milligrams of zinc gluconate daily for three months, or a placebo; then the impact of the supplement on zinc levels and antioxidant activity (zinc acts as an antioxidant) was measured. It was found that zinc supplementation corrected deficiencies in zinc-needy patients, and also thwarted lipid peroxidation, a process by which free-radical products called peroxides attack cell membranes. Zinc thus had a protective effect on health.

PROBING THE POWER OF AMINO ACIDS

By definition, amino acids are linked-together pieces of protein that we get from food or that our bodies make on their own. Individual amino acids are isolated and produced as free-form amino acid supplements. You can purchase them as capsules or tablets, in powdered nutritional drinks, or in sports nutrition bars.

Amino acids have far-reaching duties in the body—from building and repairing tissue to producing chemicals that make our brains function. Supplemental amino acids have become popular for a wide range of uses. One intriguing new application of amino acid supplements is in the treatment of diabetes. Here's a rundown on three amino acids that have been researched for their role in controlling diabetes.

L-ARGININE

Arginine has a number of important functions in the body. It is essential for growing children and needed supplementally for people with liver or kidney disease. Arginine is also required to manufacture creatine, an important chemical in the muscles that provides the energy for contractions.

How Arginine May Help Control Diabetes

Although additional research is needed, arginine appears to improve the body's use of insulin and thus may be beneficial in the treatment of type 2 diabetes. In one study, intravenous doses of arginine improved insulin sensitivity in people with type 2 diabetes, as well as those who were obese. No one yet knows whether oral supplements of arginine confer the same benefit.

Though limited, current knowledge about arginine and diabetes suggests that this potentially helpful supplement represents an avenue of research clearly worth pursuing.

Brown rice, nuts, seeds, and whole grains are high in arginine.

L-CARNITINE

Carnitine is an amino acid–like nutrient found in every cell in our bodies but concentrated mostly in muscle tissue. Smaller amounts are distributed in the blood, liver, kidneys, and brain. Foods containing carnitine include meat, nuts, dairy products, and whole grains.

Carnitine's major role in the body is to shovel fat into the cells' mitochondria (cellular furnaces) to be broken down for energy. Because of this, carnitine has a reputation as a fat burner, but few studies have supported a fat-burning benefit for this nutrient.

How Carnitine May Help Control Diabetes

Supplemental carnitine may help make cells more sensitive to insulin and less likely to resist it. That's the conclusion of several studies, which found that intravenous doses of carnitine (1–4 grams daily) reduced insulin resistance. One caveat: It is not yet known whether oral tablets or capsules of carnitine can do the same.

Supplemental carnitine is also being researched for its role in treating heart disease, so it may be of some value in preventing dreaded heart-related complications. In addition, carnitine supplementation has been used to enhance muscle strength and energy in dialysis patients. It also improves blood flow and nerve function in patients with diabetes.

L-TAURINE

Taurine is a building block of all other amino acids. It is highly concentrated in the heart muscle, white blood cells, muscles, and the central nervous system. Your body needs taurine to properly utilize sodium, potassium, calcium, and magnesium. Taurine prevents the depletion of potassium from the heart muscle and thus helps prevent the development of irregular heartbeats. This amino acid also protects nerve cells in the brain against free-radical damage, oxygen loss, and toxins.

All animal foods are rich in taurine.

How Taurine May Help Control Diabetes

As a treatment for diabetes, taurine has been studied only in animals. Results of these studies show that taurine may help normalize blood glucose levels, improve the body's use of insulin, and reduce abdominal fat. Writing in a 2000 issue of *Alternative Medicine Review*, Gregory S. Kelly, N.D., noted: "While it is impossible to extrapolate these results to human subjects, this research does suggest taurine is a nutritional intervention that merits further investigation."

FRIENDLY FATS

Think about it: On most healthy diets, you're advised to "cut the fat." But what if you were told to "up the fat"? Without feeling guilty, you can do just that—particularly if that fat comes in the form of one of the three supplements described below.

CONJUGATED LINOLEIC ACID (CLA)

Conjugated linoleic acid (CLA) is a body-friendly fat that provides excellent health insurance against a variety of ills, including obesity, diabetic complications such as heart disease, even diabetes itself. CLA is a naturally occurring fatty acid present in dairy products (most notably, milk fat) as well as in meat, sunflower oil, and safflower oil. It is formed when the bacteria in a cow's gut break down the essential fatty acid, linoleic acid, in the corn and soybeans the animal eats. CLA is available as a dietary supplement.

How CLA May Help Control Diabetes

CLA may be beneficial in treating diabetes for at least three reasons. Reason one: It appears to control blood glucose levels. One study involving prediabetic rats found that CLA reduced too-high levels of glucose in the blood. The researchers feel that CLA might turn out to be an important therapy for the prevention and treatment of type 2 diabetes.

Reason two: Much research with animals and humans documents that CLA is a potent fat fighter. That's important, particularly if you have type 2 diabetes and are struggling with your weight. In tests with mice, CLA pared down body fat (even at night), curbed appetite, boosted metabolism—and spot-reduced the animals' abdominal area!

Although the mechanism of CLA's fat-fighting action is unclear, researchers have found that it encourages the breakdown of fat, stifles a fat storage enzyme called *lipoprotein lipase*, and kills off fat cells. All three factors could be responsible for CLA's fat-burning benefits—at least in animals.

But what about in humans? A string of new evidence from human trials shows that while CLA will not decrease your body weight, it does something better: It reduces body fat and builds body-firming muscle.

Reason three: CLA may help prevent heart disease. In experimental animals, CLA thwarted the formation of plaque, the fatty deposits in and on the lining of the artery walls that lead to atherosclerosis. What's more, animals fed CLA have significantly reduced levels of low-density cholesterol, very-low-density cholesterol, and triglycerides—three nasty conspirators in heart disease.

EVENING PRIMROSE OIL

Evening primrose oil comes from a plant that grows wild along roadsides. It is so named because its yellow flowers resemble in color real primroses, and these flowers open only in the evening.

Extracted from the seeds of the plant, evening primrose oil is a rich source of various essential fatty acids, which protect the integrity of cell walls, help remove cholesterol and other fats from the body, and produce hormonelike substances called prostaglandins. Prostaglandins regulate nearly every system in your body, including your cardiovascular, immune, endocrine, central nervous, digestive, and reproductive systems.

How Evening Primrose Oil May Help Control Diabetes

Evening primrose oil has long been used as an alternative treatment for diabetes. One reason is that people with diabetes are often deficient in a special enzyme called desaturase, which is responsible for building many important components in the body. Without this enzyme, the body cannot convert an essential fatty acid called linolenic acid into another type of fatty acid called gamma-linolenic acid (GLA). GLA is involved in producing beneficial prostaglandins, which reduce inflammation, dilate blood vessels, and inhibit abnormal blood clotting.

The impairment of such a critical enzyme creates a deficiency in essential fatty acid metabolism, which in turn leads to diabetic complications, primarily poor nerve conduction and sluggish blood flow in the extremities.

Evening primrose oil is rich in GLA. That's a plus because GLA does not require desaturase for breakdown by the body. Thus, some alternative care practitioners believe that supplementation with evening primrose oil can supply needed amounts of

GLA, circumvent an essential fatty acid deficiency, and thus help prevent diabetic complications.

Most of the research supporting this view has been conducted with animals, but the results are promising. Nearly all of the studies have found that evening primrose oil corrects impaired nerve conduction and poor blood flow.

FISH OIL

Nutritional mystery: Why do Eskimos get diabetes at much lower rates than their genetic cousins, the Pima Indians of southern Arizona? In a word, fish.

Sleuthing scientists think that because Eskimos eat a lot of fish and Pima Indians rarely eat it, the fatty acids in fish somehow prevent diabetes. Indeed, research upholds this link. One study of people age forty and older found that those who ate salmon (a fatty fish) every day had a 50 percent lower chance of developing glucose intolerance than those who seldom ate fish. Some researchers believe that fatty acids in fish may enhance the delivery of glucose into cells.

Which brings up the question: Are fish oil supplements beneficial in treating diabetes, particularly if you're not a fish eater? Let's look at some of the evidence.

How Fish Oil Supplements May Help Control Diabetes

Scientists have discovered that certain types of oils from fish and shellfish, called omega-3 fatty acids, have protective benefits against a trio of cardiovascular problems: heart disease, stroke, and abnormal blood clotting. One factor in the development of these conditions is an excess of triglycerides in the bloodstream. People with type 2 diabetes sometimes have higher levels of triglycerides and cholesterol because the liver more readily converts carbohydrates into fats (including triglycerides). Omega-3 fatty acids appear to counteract this conversion and thus have a beneficial effect on triglyceride levels.

The medical evidence that fish oil lowers triglycerides is fairly firm. But here's a red flag: A Mayo Clinic statistical study, called a meta-analysis, of about twenty-one trials involving people with type 2 diabetes found that while fish oil doses (3–18 grams daily) slashed triglyceride levels, they unfortunately raised levels of harmful LDL cholesterol, particularly in individuals who used the higher doses.

On a more positive note: Fish oil may improve insulin action. One study found that fish oil (15 grams daily) along with vitamin E (200 milligrams daily) for ten weeks improved insulin resistance.

Taken during pregnancy, cod liver oil, a specific type of fish oil, may prevent a child from developing type 1 diabetes. That's the finding of a study conducted in Norway in which women who took cod liver oil during pregnancy reduced by 66 percent the chances of their kids becoming diabetic.

HERBAL HELPERS

The use of plants to treat diabetes is a centuries-old practice, dating back to ancient Egyptian physicians in 1550 B.C. who recommended a high-fiber diet of wheat grains as a remedy for the disease. The oral diabetes drug metformin (Glucophage) originated from goat's rue or French lilac, an herb used to treat diabetes since medieval times. Metformin is the only diabetes drug that has its origins from a botanical source. Worldwide, more than four hundred herbal remedies have been documented for managing diabetes, and in many cultures herbs are an accepted part of treatment for the disease.

Although hundreds of herbs have been used to treat diabetes, only a handful have been scientifically studied for their effectiveness. Some of the better-studied herbs are discussed below.

BILBERRY (*Vaccinium Myrtillus*)

Bilberry is the European version of the American blueberry. Although commonly used in pies and jellies, bilberry has become an important medicinal herb worldwide. As an herbal supplement, bilberry is sold as an extract, meaning that the herb that has been broken down or processed so that its active ingredients can be used in the product.

Extracts of bilberry contain disease-fighting antioxidants that help protect cells in the walls of the capillaries and increases their flexibility. This allows more oxygen-carrying red blood cells to reach the tissues. Also, the extract stimulates new capillary formation. Together, these actions suggest that bilberry extract may strengthen capillaries in tissues such as the retina. Bilberry also has proved to be beneficial in treating hardening of the arteries, or atherosclerosis. The extract appears to prevent plaque from building up in the arteries.

How Bilberry May Help Control Diabetes

Usually, the fruit of the plant is used in herbal supplements. But before the availability of insulin, the leaves were used as a treatment for diabetes because they contain an active ingredient called neomyrtillin. In research with people with type 2 diabetes, neomyrtillin has been shown to lower glucose levels following a meal. Neomyrtillin has also been found to enhance the glucose-lowering effect of insulin and reduce insulin requirements.

In addition, bilberry is rich in the mineral chromium, which is thought to be responsible for its antidiabetic effect.

CINNAMON (*Cinnamomum Verum*)

Cinnamon is derived from the bark of a tree of the laurel family. In addition to spicing up foods, cinnamon has been approved by the German Commission E to ease nausea, relieve stomach gas, and treat the loss of appetite. (Commission E is Germany's equivalent of our Food and Drug Administration.)

How Cinnamon May Help Control Diabetes

More than a decade ago, researchers at the Beltsville (Maryland) Human Nutrition Research Center began analyzing various plants and spices used in folk medicine. They discovered that a few spices—most notably cinnamon—made fat cells more responsive to insulin.

With subsequent experiments, the researchers isolated cinnamon's most active compound—methylhydroxy chalcone polymer (MHCP)—and found that it increased the conversion of glucose to energy by twenty times in a test tube experiment with fat cells. Another plus for MHCP: It blocked the formation of dangerous free radicals. Squelching free-radical activity can reduce or slow the progression of diabetic complications.

The researchers tested forty-nine other plant extracts, including extracts from witch hazel, green and black teas, allspice, basil, bay leaves, cloves, sage, flaxseed meal, and mushrooms. But none compared to MHCP's effect on glucose metabolism, even though some of the herbs—tea, flaxseed meal, and basil—have been reported to be effective antidiabetic agents.

COROSOLIC ACID

It doesn't yet have top billing as a natural remedy for diabetes, but corosolic acid is a rising star. This little-known supplement may have a health-saving role to play in the future for controlling diabetes and preventing some of its complications.

Corosolic acid is an extract of the leaves of the banaba plant (*Lagerstroemia speciosa*), grown in the Philippines and other parts of Asia. In these areas of the world, the banaba plant boasts a long history of use as a folk medicine, with many benefits that have been verified by scientific studies. One of these benefits is that corosolic acid reduces the accumulation of triglycerides, a blood fat that, in excessive amounts, can contribute to heart disease.

How Corosolic Acid May Help Control Diabetes

Studies with animals suggest that corosolic acid acts like insulin to ease glucose into cells and thus reduce glucose in the blood. In fact, corosolic acid has been described as a *phytoinsulin*, or plant insulin. Corsolic acid may reduce glycation as well.

If it can do all this, plus reduce triglycerides, so much the better. Some people with diabetes have high triglycerides and are thus at high risk for complications such as heart disease, high blood pressure, and stroke. Corosolic acid might deliver a one-two punch against the disease by helping patients control glucose and maintain more favorable levels of blood fats.

FENUGREEK (*Trigonella Foenumgraecum*)

Cultivated throughout the Mediterranean region, the fenugreek plant produces seeds that have long history of use as a restorative remedy, particularly to treat loss of appetite, digestive problems, and inflammation of the skin. When taken internally, fenugreek reduces blood sugar, increases lactation, and enhances wound healing. The seeds are rich in fiber, saponins (plant chemicals that contain carbohydrate molecules), and protein. The part of the seed rich in fiber is thought to be partly responsible for the herb's blood sugar-lowering effect. The seed also contains an active compound called trigonelline, which acts as a blood sugar–lowering agent.

How Fenugreek May Help Control Diabetes

As an antidiabetic herb, fenugreek has been studied in people with type 1 and type 2 diabetes. In one experiment involving people with type 1 diabetes, researchers in India tested the effects of defatted fenugreek seed powder (100 grams), divided into two equal doses and incorporated into the patients' diet. A control group followed a diet without the fenugreek seed.

By the end of the ten-day experiment, the fenugreek-supplemented group showed significantly reduced fasting blood glucose levels and improved glucose tolerance. LDL cholesterol, VLDL cholesterol, and triglycerides had dropped significantly too. The researchers concluded that fenugreek seeds are useful in the management of diabetes.

In people with type 2 diabetes, researchers in Israel found that powdered fenugreek seeds (15 grams daily) significantly reduced blood glucose levels following meals. They noted that fenugreek may have potential benefit in treating type 2 diabetes.

GARLIC (*Allium Sativum*)

This centuries-old remedy may have preventive and curative properties in a wide range of ailments, including heart disease, cancer, immune system disorders, and possibly diabetes. The cloves and oil of garlic contain more than two hundred biologically active compounds that appear to positively alter the course of many illnesses. Cultivated worldwide, garlic has been used as a dietary supplement for the treatment of diabetes in Asia, Europe, and the Middle East.

How Garlic May Help Control Diabetes

Most of the studies on garlic's antidiabetic effect have been conducted with animals. In two of these studies, an active ingredient in garlic (S-allylcysteine sulfoxide) improved diabetes in rats better than treatment with glyburide (an oral diabetes drug) or insulin did. Researchers theorized that garlic may increase insulin secretion from the beta cells of the pancreas.

Although garlic appears to work in diabetic laboratory animals, it's not working as well in humans. The only human study, which involved people with type 2 diabetes, failed to show any effect of garlic on lowering glucose levels. Garlic has however, been proved to reduce cholesterol and help prevent heart disease, a widespread complication of diabetes.

GINSENG

Used for thousands of years in the Orient as a tonic to strengthen and restore health, ginseng is one of the most popular herbal remedies in use today. It comes from the root of a medicinal plant in the ginseng family (Araliaceae), and there are several varieties. *Panax ginseng* is the Asian variety, also known as true ginseng or Chinese or Korean ginseng. It grows in the mountainous forests of eastern Asia and is the most widely used form of ginseng. *Panax quinquefolis,* or American ginseng, is found in the woodlands of the eastern and central United States and Canada. *Eleutherococcus senticosus* goes by various names: Siberian ginseng, Russian ginseng, eleuthero, or in China, ciwujia. It grows in Siberia, China, and

Korea. Although part of the Araliaceae family, eleuthero is not a member of the *Panax* species. Eleuthero, however, has medicinal properties and actions similar to those of other ginsengs.

Panax ginseng and eleuthero are approved medicines in Germany. In fact, the German Commission E states that these ginsengs can be used "as a tonic for invigoration and fortification in times of fatigue and debility, for declining capacity for work and concentration, also during convalescence."

How Ginseng May Help Control Diabetes

All three major varieties of ginseng have been studied to some degree for their role in controlling diabetes. The most intriguing study was published in 2000. Researchers at the University of Toronto found that American ginseng lowered blood sugar levels by 20 percent in patients with type 2 diabetes when 3 grams of the herb were taken forty minutes before a meal. This was the first clinical trial to demonstrate the effect of American ginseng on blood glucose levels in humans. Previous studies with rodents found that American ginseng, *Panax ginseng*, and eleuthero all have significant blood sugar–lowering properties.

More proof of an antidiabetic effect: In an eight-week study conducted in 1995, ginseng (200 milligrams daily) improved glycated hemoglobin, reduced fasting blood glucose, promoted weight loss, and enhanced mood in patients with type 2 diabetes. It is not clear from the published study which type of ginseng was used, however.

GYMNEMA SILVESTRE

Gymnema silvestre is an herb derived from the leaves of a tree native to Africa and India. It is a member of the botanical family Asclepiadaceae, named after the Greek god of healing, Asclepius.

Gymnema is best known for its ability to abolish the sensation of sweetness. In fact, the Hindu name for this herb is gurmar, which means "sugar killer." So if you're a sucker for sugar, this herb may curb your cravings by interfering with the ability to taste sweetness. The active ingredient in gymnema, gymnemic acid, has been shown to block sugar absorption in the body.

How Gymnema May Help Control Diabetes

Gymnema has long been used in India and Asia to help treat diabetes, and several modern studies show that it can boost the production and activity of insulin, reduce blood sugar levels, and lower levels of blood fats.

In a 1990 study, when twenty-seven people with type 1 diabetes on insulin therapy took 400 milligrams a day of a gymnema extract, the outcome was fascinating. Supplementing with the herb reduced the patients' insulin requirements, lowered their glycated hemoglobin, and normalized blood fats.

How did gymnema work such wonders? Researchers speculate that the herb enhances the action of supplemental insulin, possibly by regenerating or revitalizing beta cells in the pancreas. This explanation is based on an animal study, in which extracts obtained from the leaves of gymnema doubled the number of islet and beta cells in the pancreas of diabetic rats.

MILK THISTLE (*Silybum Marianum*)

The milk thistle plant is endowed with a compound called silymarin, which is revered as a liver tonic in India's five-thousand-year-old Ayurvedic system of medicine. Milk thistle and silymarin are German Commission E–approved medicines for treating liver disease. Silymarin is also used to treat loss of appetite and gallbladder problems.

How Milk Thistle May Help Control Diabetes

Recent studies have suggested that silymarin may help fight type 2 diabetes by reducing insulin resistance. Silymarin is rich in antioxidants, which may exert an antidiabetic effect by defusing free-radical attacks on cells.

The results of one study of sixty people with type 2 diabetes point to the promise of silymarin in treating the disease. In this study, all the patients had been receiving insulin therapy for at least two years and suffered from alcohol-induced liver damage (cirrhosis).

For one year, half the group supplemented with 600 milligrams of silymarin, along with their standard therapy; the other half remained on standard therapy only. By the end of the year, the silymarin-treated patients experienced several benefits.

Benefit one: Three important measurements improved. Their average daily glucose levels fell from 202 mg/dl to 172 mg/dl, their glycated hemoglobin levels decreased significantly, and their average daily insulin requirement dropped as well.

Benefit two: The silymarin-treated patients did not have any increase in the number of mild or severe hypoglycemic reactions. This suggests that silymarin stabilized as well as lowered their blood glucose levels.

Benefit three: Their liver function improved.

None of these benefits was experienced by the patients in the standard therapy group.

DESIGNING A SUPPLEMENT PROGRAM

Most of the supplemental nutrients, including vitamins and minerals, you need to control your diabetes and discourage its complications can be obtained from an antioxidant formula, taken once daily. For added protection and with your doctor's blessing, you may want to take additional vitamin C and vitamin E, along with the other antidiabetic antioxidants, alpha-lipoic acid, and coenzyme Q10.

As for minerals, you can generally get protective levels of these minerals from food and from supplements, with the exception of calcium and magnesium. Once-a-day antioxidant formulas are often low in these minerals because both are bulky and make the pill too large. Therefore, you may want to supplement with extra calcium and magnesium, as long your doctor okays it.

Do not supplement with isolated amino acids for longer than a few weeks at a time, since excess amino acids in your system may place an undue burden on the work of your kidneys. The exception to this is carnitine, which is very safe and has no known side effects.

Supplemental fats are generally safe, but you should first talk to your doctor and dietitian about using them. Regarding fish oil supplements: You can get the same protection supplements afford by eating two to three fish or shellfish meals each week.

Most of the herbs under investigation for treating diabetes are relatively safe. Even so, herbs are a form of medicine. Just because an herb may have some antidiabetic effects, you should not self-prescribe that herb unless first checking with your physician and health-care team.

Most of the supplements discussed can be used concurrently, particularly antioxidants, B complex vitamins, minerals, and fat supplements. However, be careful about taking a handful of different products, particularly amino acids and herbs at the same time. It's unclear how well some combinations work. They may enhance the effects of each other; they also may not. If you notice any untoward reaction after taking supplements, check with your doctor.

With herbs in particular, it's better to try one supplement or one product at a time. Then, give each herb a trial period before deciding whether it's helping you.

In the box opposite, you'll find a suggested supplement program. A reminder: Always get your physician's approval before taking dietary and herbal supplements.

・・・

WHAT THE EXPERTS ADVISE
Top-Ten Strategies for Using Natural Remedies
Kathleen Head, N.D.

Kathleen Head, N.D., is a nationally recognized naturopathic physician and the author of *The Natural Pharmacist: Everything You Need to Know About Diabetes* (1999), *Natural Treatments for Diabetes* (2000), and *The Natural Pharmacist: Support for Diabetes* (2001). Dr. Head is a senior editor of the peer-reviewed Medline-indexed journal *Alternative Medicine Review*. Here are her tips for controlling diabetes with natural remedies.

1. The most important aspect of controlling diabetes and preventing the associated complications, no matter what methods are used for blood sugar control, is frequent (several times daily) checking of blood sugar.

2. Pay close attention to how particular foods affect your blood sugar. Ideal diets vary from person to person, but the most important factor is eating a wide variety of fresh vegetables of as many different colors as possible. High-quality protein should include fish, lean meat, poultry, eggs, tofu, and/or legumes. Meat and produce should be organic whenever possible.

3. People with diabetes tend to have deficiencies of a number of vitamins and minerals. The basis of a good sup-

A SUGGESTED SUPPLEMENT PROGRAM

ANTIOXIDANTS	RECOMMENDED RANGE/DOSAGE
An antioxidant vitamin/mineral supplement (choose a supplement made by a pharmaceutical company or other reputable manufacturer)	Once daily
Vitamin C	500 mg daily
Vitamin E	200–800 mg daily, depending on doctor's recommendation
Alpha-lipoic acid	600–800 mg daily
Coenzyme Q10	30–60 mg daily
B COMPLEX VITAMINS	**RECOMMENDED RANGE/DOSAGE**
With the exception of biotin, additional B-vitamins can be obtained from an antioxidant vitamin/mineral formula.	Once daily (antioxidant formula); 200–400 mg daily of biotin
MINERALS	**RECOMMENDED RANGE/DOSAGE**
Calcium	1,000 mg daily (men and women, ages nineteen to fifty); 1,200 mg daily (men and women, ages fifty-one to seventy and over)
Chromium	50–200 mcg daily. You can obtain this amount from your antioxidant formula, which contains 150 mcg chromium, on average.
Magnesium	320 mg daily (women); 420 mg daily (men). Antioxidant formulas generally contain about 100 mg.
Potassium	Antioxidant formulas generally contain about 10 mg. Check with your doctor prior to taking high doses.

A SUGGESTED SUPPLEMENT PROGRAM (cont'd)

Vanadium	10–60 mcg daily, which can usually be obtained from food. Antioxidant formulas contain about 10 mg.
Zinc	12 mg (women); 15 mg (men). To improve glucose metabolism, some health-care practitioners recommend 15–25 mg a day of zinc. Antioxidant formulas contain about 15 mg.
AMINO ACIDS	**RECOMMENDED RANGE/DOSAGE**
L-arginine	None yet identified
L-carnitine or acetyl-l-carnitine	Optimum oral dose not yet identified
L-taurine	None yet identified
FAT SUPPLEMENTS	**RECOMMENDED RANGE/DOSAGE**
Conjugated linoleic acid (CLA)	2–4 g daily
Evening primrose oil	2–4 g daily
Fish oil	None yet identified
HERBS	**RECOMMENDED RANGE/DOSAGE**
Bilberry	None yet identified
Corosolic acid	Available in supplements designed to control blood glucose levels
Fenugreek	25–50 g daily (as seed powder mixed in food or water)
Garlic	None yet identified
Ginseng	200 mg daily
Gymnema sylvestre	400 mg daily; ¾ teaspoon in a cup of boiling water for tea
Milk thistle	200–600 mg daily

plement plan should be a high-potency multiple vitamin-mineral formula in capsules.

4. Essential fatty acids, particularly GLA, help prevent several complications of high blood sugar, including nerve damage (neuropathy), kidney problems, and heart disease. Sources of GLA include black currant, borage, and evening primrose oils.

5. Antioxidants are very important, since many of the complications of diabetes have been associated with free-radical damage. One of the best is alpha-lipoic acid, and there are some good research studies supporting its use, especially for prevention of neuropathy. Vitamin E is important for prevention of heart disease and retinopathy.

6. Extracts of bilberry, from the blueberry family, contain potent antioxidant flavonoids that have been found to strengthen the blood vessels in the eye and may prevent retinal damage.

7. Bioflavonoids and vitamin C can prevent formation of molecules called polyols that accumulate in cells that are exposed to high amounts of sugar. Polyols are the culprits involved in sugar cataracts and other complications of diabetes. Quercetin is one of the most potent of these bioflavonoids. It is found in cabbage, garlic, grapefruit, onions, and other plant foods.

8. Water-soluble fiber helps normalize blood sugar and should be taken with meals to slow the absorption of sugar from the meal. Fibers in this category include defatted fenugreek powder and legumes (beans, lentils, peas).

9. Minimize stress as much as possible since stress can adversely affect blood sugar. This may be easier said than done, but a regular practice of exercise, meditation, yoga, or

some other relaxation activity is recommended. Support and understanding from loved ones also goes a long way toward minimizing stress.

10. Several vitamins, minerals, and herbs can help lower blood sugar, including chromium, vanadium, biotin, and gymnema. In the case of type 1 diabetes, insulin will always be required, but the supplements may help to decrease the amount of insulin that is needed by making the insulin work more efficiently. For type 2, one or more of the supplements, along with exercise, weight loss, and dietary changes, may either keep blood sugar normal without other medication or help medication work more effectively.

STEP THREE

Test Your Blood Sugar Regularly

Keeping tabs on your blood sugar is one of the most important actions you can take to control your diabetes and keep it from getting worse. Termed *self-monitoring of blood glucose*, or *SMBG* for short, blood sugar testing is an easy, convenient way to tell how much glucose is in your bloodstream. Best of all, there's no need to show up at your doctor's office for the test. You can do it at home with a special kit.

Before at-home self-monitoring kits were available, people with diabetes had to test their urine to learn if their diabetes was under control (which wasn't very accurate), or they had to have their glucose tested at the doctor's office every few months. The results were sent to the lab and were not available until days later. Because blood sugar can waver so much from day to day, the results were largely irrelevant.

SMBG lets you know the level of your glucose any time of the day or night. You get immediate feedback on what you eat and what you do. Depending on the reading, you can adjust the amount of food you eat, the intensity of your exercise, or the amount of insulin or medication you need. You can also tell how well your efforts at controlling diabetes are working. If you're not feeling right but don't know why, checking your blood glucose level may pinpoint the problem.

More important, SMBG is vital for the prevention of long-term complications of diabetes. In the Diabetes Complications and Control Trial, the most comprehensive study of diabetes control ever, researchers found that keeping blood glucose levels close to normal helps prevent or delay complications in people with type 1 diabetes.

SMBG is thus an essential tool for achieving tighter control of your diabetes, no matter which type you have. In short, SMBG gives you a sense of mastery over your diabetes—and your life.

In this step, you'll learn about:

- What to look for when you test
- How to test
- When to test
- How to record your test results
- How to handle emergencies

WHAT TO LOOK FOR WHEN YOU TEST

When you test, you check to see whether your blood sugar falls within a desirable range. For most people with diabetes, ideal ranges are:

- Before meals: 80–120 mg/dl
- At bedtime: 100–140 mg/dl

Your health care team may set additional goals for you, and these may include:

- One hour after a meal: 90–150 mg/dl
- Two hours after a meal: 80–140 mg/dl

HOW TO TEST YOUR BLOOD

SMBG is very easy, thanks to the availability of new testing tools. Currently, there are two ways to perform SMBG: the finger-stick test, which is more accurate; and a noninvasive device called the GlucoWatch, which sends a small electric current over the skin, stimulating the secretion of a tiny bit of fluid. The GlucoWatch is great if you don't like needles.

The Finger-Stick Test

To do this test, prick your finger with a special needle (called a *lancet*) to obtain a drop of blood. There are different types of lancets available, and they vary in size and shape. You'll have to experiment with the type that works best for you and feels the least painful. Always use your own lancet; don't borrow used lancets, or you could risk infection with a blood-borne disease.

Prick your finger as superficially as possible, without going too deep. Each time you prick, try to rotate the puncture sites on your fingers to minimize damage. Try the sides of your fingertips, as well as the central parts. Use your thumbs as an alternate location too.

Place the blood drop on a test strip and wait for the strip to change color. The amount of glucose in the blood activates the color change. Next, match the color of the strip to a color chart on the test-strip container. The colors on the chart represent ranges of glucose levels.

Another way to test the blood drop is to use a glucose meter, a special device that reads your test strip. With some meters, you place the drop of blood on a test strip, wait for the strip to develop, wipe off the blood, and place the strip in the meter. With other meters, you simply place the blood drop in the meter and wait for the results. Both types of meters display your blood glucose level on a screen.

Blood glucose meters are highly accurate. However, certain matters of human error can produce incorrect readings. To prevent this from happening:

- Keep your meter clean.
- Keep your meter at room temperature; do not expose it to extremes of temperature.
- Use a blood drop that's large enough.
- Don't use outdated test strips.
- Ask your health care team to observe your testing skills every so often.

The GlucoWatch

Worn on the wrist like a watch, the GlucoWatch measures glucose collected through the skin, not the blood. It measures and displays glucose levels automatically, as often as every twenty minutes for up to twelve hours, by sending tiny electric currents through the skin. The device also stores information that can be retrieved at the touch of a button and used to track trends. In addition, the device has an alarm that goes off if blood sugar is too high or too low. GlucoWatch is FDA-approved and requires a prescription. You can learn more about the GlucoWatch at the manufacturer's Web site: www.cygn.com.

Be sure to work closely with your health care team to assess which monitoring systems, including the GlucoWatch, are appropriate for your personal situation.

WHEN TO TEST

If you have type 1 diabetes, your doctor will want you to test your blood four to five times each day. Research shows that when people test several times a day, they achieve better glucose control.

With type 2 diabetes, you don't need to test your blood quite as often, because blood glucose levels stay fairly stable throughout the day. Usually, people with type 2 diabetes who are not taking medication may have to test once, twice, or three times a day. Testing once a day at the same time each day is the absolute minimum.

If you're taking an oral diabetes agent, you may have to test more frequently to help your doctor determine the most effective dose and to monitor how well the medication is working. Medications should not be adjusted unless you're performing SMBG on a regular basis.

There are no hard-and-fast rules on when to test. But, according to most diabetes experts, there are standard times to test, particularly if you're looking for patterns in the rise and fall of your glucose levels:

- Before breakfast, lunch, dinner, and large snacks, every day
- Before bedtime, every day
- One to two hours after breakfast, lunch, dinner, and large snacks, occasionally
- Before and after exercise
- At 2 A.M. or 3 A.M. about once a week

RECORD YOUR RESULTS

After testing your blood, write down the results, along with the date and time. You can obtain a special log from your doctor or at most drugstores.

In addition, record any related events, such as stress, illness, or exercise, that may have influenced your blood glucose levels. This log can help you, your doctor, and other members of your health care team track how well you're controlling your diabetes. By reviewing your log, your health care team can also analyze swings in your blood sugar and adjust your diet, exercise, and medication accordingly, if necessary.

Some important advice: The results of your blood sugar tests can evoke feelings of anger, frustration, confusion, and depression if the ranges aren't as expected. Do not judge yourself negatively as a result of the numbers. Keep in mind that your blood sugar levels are a way to track how well you're controlling your diabetes. The results indicate that you may need to alter your self-care plan, or, better yet, stay the course.

HANDLING EMERGENCIES

Testing your blood sugar regularly is also an important way to avert three serious yet preventable short-term problems: *hypoglycemia*, *hyperglycemia*, and *ketoacidosis*. All three represent potential emergencies, so it's important to be alert to their warning signs and how to deal with them.

Hypoglycemia

Hypoglycemia—a lower-than-normal concentration of glucose in the blood—can develop if you are taking insulin, eating too little, exercising too hard or too long, experiencing stress, or drinking alcohol on an empty stomach. With type 1 diabetes, you may have one or two episodes of hypoglycemia a week, on average. Hypoglycemia is much less common if you have type 2 diabetes.

Hypoglycemia produces these symptoms:

- Shakiness
- Hunger
- Nervousness
- Fatigue
- Headache
- Confusion
- Dizziness
- Rapid heartbeat

You should always be prepared for a hypoglycemic reaction (also commonly known as an *insulin reaction* if you are taking insulin). Generally, hypoglycemia can occur if your blood sugar drops below 50 mg/dl. Some people, however, may become hypoglycemic at levels higher than 50 mg/dl.

Consuming something that contains 15 grams of carbohydrate will usually alleviate the symptoms of hypoglycemia. Here are some examples recommended by the American Diabetes Association:

½ cup (⅓ can) of a regular soft drink
½ cup of fruit juice
1 cup of skim milk
2 tablespoons of raisins
3 hard candies
1 tablespoon of sugar

In addition to these quick-acting carbohydrates, there are over-the-counter products you can buy to treat hypoglycemia. Called *reaction-products*, they include flavored glucose tablets or gels and are available in pharmacies. It's a good idea to keep these on hand, just in case you need them.

If hypoglycemia is not resolved, it can lead to unconsciousness or convulsions. So if you're diabetic and use insulin, make family members, friends, and coworkers aware of the fact that you take the drug. Further, they should know how to take care of you in the event of an insulin reaction. According to the American Diabetes Association, they should do the following if you become unconscious:

- Summon emergency help.
- Administer an injection of another hormone, glucagon, which opposes the action of insulin.
- Do *not* administer insulin.
- Do *not* give you food or fluids or put their hands in your mouth.

Hyperglycemia

When blood glucose levels soar to levels higher than 250 mg/dl, a condition called hyperglycemia results. With type 1 diabetes, it is usually caused by having too little insulin in your body. Hyperglycemia can occur in type 2 diabetes, but is less common. Even so, it is crucial to know the warning signs:

- Headache
- Blurry vision
- Extreme thirst
- Frequent need to urinate
- Dry, itchy skin.

Ignoring hyperglycemia can lead to a serious, but preventable, emergency called ketoacidosis.

Ketoacidosis

More common in type 1 diabetes than in type 2, ketoacidosis is the result of excessively high glucose levels in your blood, triggered by overeating or treating yourself with an insufficient dose of insulin. Sickness or stress can cause overly elevated glucose too.

Whatever the reason for ketoacidosis, the bottom line is that you have too little insulin in your system. As a result, your body starts breaking down fat for energy. The by-products of this process are dangerous chemicals called *ketones*, detectable in urine. Ketones are a warning sign that your body is burning fat, rather than glucose, for fuel. They also indicate that your diabetes may be out of control.

Ketoacidosis can produce the following symptoms:

- Vomiting
- Stomach pains
- Loss of appetite
- Fever
- Breathing problems
- Excessive thirst
- Dry, itchy skin
- Weakness
- Sleepiness
- Blurry vision
- Fruity breath odor
- Dry mouth
- Frequent urination

You can prevent ketoacidosis by testing your urine for ketones with special test kits available at pharmacies, as well as by testing your glucose level. (Some ketone strips test for both ketones and glucose.) Urine tests come in tapes, tablets, and test strips. Although testing methods vary according to the product, here are the steps normally involved in testing urine for ketones:

- Obtain a sample of your urine in a clean container.
- Place a test strip (or other testing medium) in the sample.
- Remove the strip and shake off the excess urine.
- Wait for the test strip to change color.
- Compare the strip to a color chart that comes with the product. The chart provides a range indicating the level of ketones in your urine.
- Write down your results.

You should test your urine for ketones under the following conditions:

- You have symptoms of ketoacidosis.
- Your glucose levels are higher than 250 mg/dl.
- You are ill.
- You are under physical stress (such as surgery) or emotional stress.
- You are chronically tired.

If there are ketones in your urine, notify your physician immediately.

STEP FOUR

Get Fit to Fight Diabetes

By exercising, you can prevail over diabetes and reclaim your good health. Here's why: When you exercise, your body fuels the activity by extracting glucose from your blood for energy. This reduces your blood glucose levels. Not only that, exercise helps your body better handle insulin, use glucose, and transport it into cells. And the more active you are, the better you can control your weight.

There are other payoffs: Exercise may reduce or eliminate your need to take diabetes medications. Many people with type 2 diabetes find that after they start exercising, they no longer need pills. And those with type 1 diabetes discover that they require a lower dose of injectable insulin after they begin a regular exercise program. Having a exercise program that incorporates aerobic and strength training will step up the quality of your life immeasurably.

If these benefits sound appealing to you, it's time to get moving. In this step, you'll learn about how to:

- Exercise safely
- Control your blood glucose levels during exercise

- Design an aerobics and strength-training program suited to your needs
- Stick to your exercise program

FIRST THINGS FIRST: EXERCISING SAFELY

If you really want to be successful with your exercise program, please take the following advice:

- Wear a Med-Alert or diabetes identification bracelet or shoe tag, and make sure that it is visible while you are working out.
- Wear proper footwear to protect your feet. Silica gel or air midsoles, along with polyester or blend (cotton polyester) socks, will prevent blisters and keep your feet dry.
- If you have not exercised in a while, start slowly.
- Begin your exercise session with a warm-up and finish with a cooldown. The warm-up is light activity performed for five to ten minutes—walking at a slow pace, pedaling against very light resistance, slow stepping on a stair-climbing machine, and so forth. The warm-up should also include a five-minute period of light stretching. The warm-up decreases stress on your heart, lowers your blood pressure, increases blood flow to your heart, and keeps your joints and muscles limber.

Similarly, a cooldown is five to ten minutes of less vigorous activity to help your heart rate return to normal. It also removes exercise-generated waste products from your muscles and keeps blood from pooling in your legs. If blood is allowed to collect in your legs, blood pressure can drop

sharply, possibly causing dizziness. The cooldown keeps blood circulating back toward the heart.
- Keep your body well hydrated—before, during, and after exercise. Drink at least 16 ounces (2 cups) of water two to three hours before exercise. Then, drink 8 ounces (1 cup) of water immediately before exercise to make sure your body is well hydrated. During exercise, drink 7 to 10 ounces every ten to twenty minutes. After working out, replace any fluid you've lost by drinking 2 to 3 cups of water or other fluid within two hours following your exercise session.
- Avoid workouts in extremely hot or cold weather. Exercising in hot or humid weather increases the possibility of low blood sugar, while exercising in cold weather puts you at greater risk of developing cracked skin or frostbite, particularly if you have neuropathy or impaired circulation.
- If you have a muscle, tendon, ligament, or joint injury, do not exercise the affected body part. Such injuries take time to heal, but if you have diabetes, the healing time may be longer than usual, particularly if your circulation is impaired.
- Do not exercise if you have a cold, the flu, an infection, or other illness. During sickness, your blood glucose levels can rise due to the stress imposed on your body by the illness or infection. Exercising during an illness will only aggravate your condition and interfere with getting well.
- Report to your doctor any unusual symptoms that you experience during or after exercise. These include discomfort in your chest, neck, jaw, or arms; nausea; dizziness; fainting; shortness of breath; unusual pain; or vision problems.

GLUCOSE CONTROL DURING EXERCISE

Another yellow light before starting any exercise: Glucose can get out of kilter when you exercise, for a couple of reasons. To begin with, exercise can cause a drop in blood sugar levels (hypoglycemia) as working muscles extract the glucose they need for fuel. Normally, this is not much of a problem. But if you haven't eaten enough energy-providing carbohydrates prior to your workout, you could experience hypoglycemia while exercising.

By contrast, exercise can make blood sugar go way up, particularly if you begin exercising with excessively high blood glucose levels. When you work out, your liver releases stored glucose. If you have enough insulin in circulation, your muscles are able to use this released glucose for energy.

Trouble starts, though, when there is already too much glucose in circulation prior to exercising. This may signal that you don't have enough insulin in your system to match the amount of glucose in your blood. Thus, when you exercise, the glucose released from your liver makes your blood glucose soar even higher.

Other metabolic problems can arise during exercise. With exercise, your body burns both glucose and fat for fuel. When your body burns fat, acidic by-products of fat breakdown called ketones are produced. As long as there is enough insulin in the blood, your muscles will burn some of these ketones as an alternate fuel. But with a shortage of insulin, ketones will pile up in the blood. If ketones build up to a certain level, some will spill over into your urine. When ketones are detectable in urine, it is a warning that your body doesn't have enough insulin available to usher glucose into cells. This can occur in anyone with diabetes, but is more apt to happen if you have type 1 diabetes.

Thus, insufficient levels of insulin during exercise increase ketones and blood glucose levels. Excess glucose can spill over into your urine too. As a result, your body starts making more urine, and you get dehydrated. Dehydration, coupled with excess ketones, can cause ketoacidosis, a life-threatening condition that upsets the body's equilibrium between acid and base concentrations in bodily fluids. Ketoacidosis can subside within hours or a few days, but it is better to head it off before it begins. (For more information on ketoacidosis, see Step 4.)

To avoid ketoacidosis and blood sugar highs and lows, you must closely track glucose and ketones so you can make the proper adjustments in insulin and/or diet. Here are some important exercise precautions to take to prevent exercise-induced problems:

- Eat a well-balanced meal about two to three hours prior to exercise.
- Self-monitor your glucose levels prior to exercise. If your blood glucose is lower than 100 mg/dl, eat 15 to 20 grams of carbohydrate fifteen to thirty minutes before exercising.
- If your blood glucose is greater than 250 mg/dl, test your urine for ketones. If ketones are positive, do not exercise. Notify your doctor. If ketones are negative, proceed with your exercise session.
- Exercise with extreme caution if glucose levels are above 300 mg/dl and no ketones are present. Exercise could send your glucose levels higher, so you may want to avoid exercising until your glucose is under better control.
- Recheck your blood glucose right after exercise, or sooner if you feel any symptoms of low blood sugar. If levels are below 60 mg/dl, eat 15 to 20 grams of carbohydrate.

- If you have type 1 diabetes, monitor your blood glucose before and after exercise, and every twenty to thirty minutes during prolonged exercise.
- If you use insulin, adjust your food or insulin to accommodate your activity. Ask your doctor's advice, but adjusting insulin usually involves decreasing short-acting insulin by 30 percent prior to exercise of less than one hour; 40 percent if one to two hours; and 50 percent if exercise exceeds three hours. If you take oral diabetes drugs, you may need to alter your dosage. Check with your physician.

    Do not exercise during peak insulin time, either. With proper insulin administration, people with well-controlled type 1 diabetes will respond to exercise as well as people without diabetes.
- If you are insulin-dependent, inject insulin into less active or nonactive muscle sites. This is especially important if you have to inject insulin during exercise. Injecting a working muscle will cause a too-rapid uptake of insulin.
- Have some fast-acting glucose on hand at all times, such as glucose tablets or a glucose-electrolyte sports drink such as Gatorade.
- If blood glucose increases, test your urine for ketones. If ketones increase, avoid exercising at these increased levels of blood glucose.
- Keep a log of the response you get from each exercise session. Record your blood glucose level and the time you checked it, the amount of diabetes medication you took, the length of your workout, and the intensity of your workout. By predicting how your body responds to exercise, this log will

help you identify what to eat before and after working out, as well as how to adjust your medication dosage for future exercise sessions.

DESIGNING YOUR AEROBIC EXERCISE PROGRAM

So that you'll stick to it and reap the health rewards right away, you'll want to set up an aerobic fitness exercise program that fits you and your lifestyle. Aerobic exercise programs are generally designed around four variables: exercise choice, frequency, duration, and intensity.

Exercise Choice

It used to be that aerobics meant jogging. Not anymore. Today, there are special aerobics classes and high-tech machines, which besides their primary heart-pumping action provide muscle-toning stimulation to specific parts of the body.

For most people with diabetes, however, walking is the most commonly recommended form of aerobic activity. It's an easy-does-it exercise that's especially appropriate for anyone just beginning an aerobic exercise program. Indeed, walking has been dubbed the "ideal" exercise—and for good reason. It improves aerobic fitness, burns fat, helps prevent bone-crippling osteoporosis, and cuts the risk of developing coronary heart disease. In fact, research shows that walking nine miles (that's about three hours) a week on a consistent basis significantly reduces your chances of developing heart disease. What's more, walking is safe, convenient, and easy to do.

However, walking or its higher-effort counterparts—jogging and running—may not be appropriate for everyone, particularly those who have diabetic-related complications. For a list of exercises to avoid if you have complications, see the box on page 183.

Fortunately, though, there are many other forms of aerobic activity from which to choose. These include swimming, aquatic exercise, and stationary bicycling. There are also fun sports such as basketball, volleyball, hiking, or racquet sports that confer aerobic benefits. Of course, the very best aerobic exercise is the one you enjoy doing—and will stick to for a lifetime.

Frequency

The number of times you exercise each week is referred to as *frequency*. The general recommendation for people with diabetes is to exercise aerobically at least three times a week. Try to work up to five times a week, in order to improve cardiovascular health and, if you have type 2 diabetes, to reduce body fat.

A word of caution: Newcomers to aerobic exercise should not start out exercising five times a week! If you do, you risk injury and burnout. Instead, start out by trying to exercise two to three times a week; then gradually build to five sessions as your aerobic capacity improves or as your schedule permits.

Some diabetes experts recommend daily workouts for people with diabetes who are taking insulin. By providing consistency, daily workouts lessen the difficulty of balancing caloric needs with insulin dosage. Of course, frequency depends on your schedule. It's not always feasible to get in five or more aerobic sessions a week.

Duration

Exercise duration refers to the length of time you spend working out. For exercising novices with diabetes, short exercise bouts of ten to fifteen minutes each time are recommended at first. As you gain strength and stamina, gradually increase your workouts to thirty minutes each session. You can also squeeze your workouts into three ten-minute sessions throughout the day. Research shows that shorter bouts, performed during the day, do just as much good—in terms of aerobic fitness and weight loss—as longer exercise sessions, and they're certainly better than doing no exercise at all.

If your goal is weight control, gradually build up to exercising aerobically for forty-five to sixty minutes each time. This maximizes your fat-burning potential and helps keep your weight in check.

Intensity

Intensity—level of effort—is equally important to improving health and fitness and preventing diabetic complications. For most people with diabetes, low- to moderate-intensity exercise is recommended.

How can you tell whether you're exercising within that range of intensity? In three different ways.

HEART RATE: Aerobic intensity can be measured by your *exercising heart rate*—how fast your heart beats while exercising. At a low intensity, you're working out at a level that's 40 to 65 percent of your maximum heart rate (MHR). Moderate intensity is 65 to 75 percent of your MHR; high intensity is 75 to 90 percent of your MHR.

MHR is expressed as 220 minus your age. For example, if you're 45 years old, your maximum heart rate is 220 − 45 = 175. If your goal is to exercise at a low to moderate intensity, your heart should reach roughly 114 beats a minute (65 percent of 175 beats per minute = .65 × 175 = 114).

To find your heart rate during exercise, take your pulse at the radial artery in either wrist or at the carotid artery to the left or right of your windpipe. Place your index and middle finger (not your thumb) lightly over the artery. Don't press too hard, particularly on the carotid artery. Too much pressure can actually slow your pulse. Count the beats for fifteen seconds; then multiply that number times 4 to get your heart rate for a minute.

RATING OF PERCEIVED EXERTION (RPE): A second method of measuring your aerobic intensity is by using a scale called the rating of perceived exertion (RPE), or the Borg Scale because it was developed by Swedish exercise physiologist Gunnar Borg.

Recommended for exercisers with diabetes, the RPE helps you regulate intensity using subjective descriptions of how hard exercise feels as you exert yourself. You make this assessment based on the following scale:

BORG'S SCALE OF PERCEIVED EXERTION	
6	No exertion at all
7	Extremely light
8	
9	Very light
10	
11	Light
12	
13	Somewhat hard
14	
15	Hard (heavy)
16	
17	Very hard
18	
19	Extremely hard
20	Maximal exertion

To use the scale, listen to your body while exercising, sense your intensity, and choose the number that best describes how hard you feel you're exercising at any given moment during your workout. Here's how to gauge your intensity:

- An RPE of 11 or less indicates low-intensity exercise. At a level of 11, you'll start building cardiovascular conditioning.
- An RPE of 12 to 14 indicates moderate intensity. You feel relatively comfortable and can carry on a conversation without losing your breath. This is an appropriate level if you're a beginner to exercise or have risk factors for cardiovascular disease.
- An RPE of 15 or higher indicates high intensity. At this range, your pulse is quite rapid, and it is difficult to talk or exercise for a long period of time. You should avoid this range because it can produce unnecessary fatigue, increase the potential for hypoglycemia, and up your odds of injury, including the risk of heart attack. If you're young and already active, exercising in the 13 to 15 range is generally safe, however.

In research, the RPE has been shown to correlate well with other methods of measuring intensity, such as heart rate monitoring. A 6, for example, represents a resting heart rate of 60, and 20 represents an exercising heart rate of 200 beats per minute.

THE TALK TEST: Perhaps the easiest and most practical way to assess your intensity is the talk test. If you can carry on a conversation while exercising, without huffing and puffing, you are probably working in the low-intensity range and not overexerting yourself. A leisurely walk is a good example of low-intensity exercise.

In the moderate-intensity range, you can still talk, but you are breathing a little faster. Brisk walking weighs in as moderate-intensity exercise.

With high-intensity exercise, your heart is pounding, and your breathing is hard. You can still talk, but only in short sentences. Examples of high-intensity exercise are running, high-impact aerobics, and a fast-paced racquet ball match.

Super-high-intensity is not being able to talk and panting hard. Athletes in competitive events such as a 100-meter dash are working at super-high intensities.

DESIGNING A STRENGTH-TRAINING PROGRAM

If you're a newcomer to strength training, the starting point is to work with a qualified personal trainer who can show you the ropes. Your trainer should also provide instruction on lifting techniques, body alignment, proper breathing, and other important points involving exercise performance.

As with aerobics, a strength-training program is designed around such factors as exercise choice, intensity, duration, and frequency. These are discussed below, with special considerations that are vital if you have diabetes.

Exercise Choice

The exercises you select depend partly on your goals. For general conditioning, you should choose about eight to ten different exercises involving your major muscle groups—legs, chest, back, shoulders, abdominals, and arms. If you have "problem areas" that need slimming, such as thighs and buttocks, add some extra exercises to hit those trouble spots. Or if you're an athlete who wants to improve upper-body strength, include shoulder and back exercises specifically designed to build strength and power.

Intensity

Intensity in weight training refers to the *load* you place on your muscles—in other words, how much weight you *can* lift. Lifting very heavy loads, or poundages, is considered high-intensity exercise. Intensity in strength training also refers to the number of repetitions you perform with a certain poundage and is described as *volume*.

Lifting a heavy weight fewer times—say, six or seven—is considered *high-intensity, low-volume training*. This is a good way to build muscular strength. Athletes with diabetes who want to increase strength might consider following high-intensity, low-volume programs.

Lifting a medium weight for eight to twelve repetitions is classified as *moderate-intensity, medium-volume training*. This is an effective way to increase muscle tone and size.

Strength training that involves light weights and many repetitions (twelve to twenty) is *low-intensity, high-volume training*. It helps build muscular endurance—the ability to repeat muscle movements over and over again without tiring out. Diabetic patients with heart disease who have their physicians' approval to lift weights are generally advised to perform moderate-intensity, medium-volume workouts, or low-intensity, high-volume workouts.

The key is to challenge your muscles to work harder each time you strength train. That means progressively upping your poundages or repetitions. Muscles adapt very quickly to stresses placed on them. For continual progress, you must increase loads, do more repetitions with the same load, or both. Increasing your effort each workout makes your muscles get firmer and stronger.

Number of Sets per Exercise

Exercises for various muscles are organized into *sets*. A set is a group of repetitions, punctuated by a rest period. A *routine* is the entire collection of exercises you do each exercise session.

Generally, you begin each exercise with a set using a very light weight with high repetitions simply to warm up a specific muscle or muscle group. On your subsequent sets, called *working sets*, you add more weight (about five to ten pounds heavier) and perform fewer repetitions as the exercise becomes harder.

Here are some guidelines for determining the number of sets per exercise:

- If you're just beginning to strength train, use only two sets (a warm-up set and a working set) per exercise and work out in this manner for four to eight weeks.
- After a month or two, increase the number of sets to three (a warm-up and two working sets). Continue training with three sets per exercise for two to three months.
- As you become stronger and more experienced, up the number of sets to four or five (the first set should always be a working set). Increasing the number of sets is another way to increase strength training intensity and further challenge your muscles.

Duration

The length of time you strength train varies according to the number of sets and exercises you perform in your routine. A beginner's routine may last only twenty minutes, whereas an advanced exerciser's routine may last forty-five minutes to an hour.

Frequency

If you're a beginner, try to strength train two to three times a week, always on nonconsecutive days to give your muscles time to repair themselves. After a few months of working out, you will be ready to do more work with weights to continue your progress. Ways to do that include performing more sets of each exercise, as well as doing more exercises. Depending on your schedule, you may also want to increase your number of training days, possibly using a *split routine*. This involves working your upper body twice a week and your lower body twice a week for a total of four training days a week.

PUT DIABETES IN REVERSE WITH THESE EASY-TO-FOLLOW ROUTINES

The following sample routines are designed to show you how easy it is to incorporate the recommended amount of activity into your weekly schedule. Three plans are included: a beginning routine, for those just beginning to exercise; an intermediate routine, for those who have been exercising for at least several weeks; and an advanced routine, for those who have been exercising successfully for several weeks and want to increase intensity.

In the beginning routine, you start out slowly, with ten to fifteen minutes of brisk walking or other aerobic-type exercise three times a week, and strength-training exercises twice a week. Each week, add ten minutes to your aerobic activity. This routine is designed to help you progress slowly but at a pace that will help build your stamina in a few short weeks.

In the intermediate routine, there is an additional but optional day of scheduled aerobic activity and three days of strength training. Another option is to perform two days of strength training and four to five days of aerobic activity.

In the advanced routine, there are four days of scheduled aerobic activity and three days of strength-training exercises. The prescribed number of sets per exercise increases. Another option is to perform two days of strength training and four to five days of aerobic activity. Of course not everyone's schedule will match these plans exactly. The plans are flexible. You can adapt them to your own schedule by mixing and matching the days on which you perform certain activities.

BEGINNING EXERCISE ROUTINE	
Sunday	Rest
Monday	Aerobics (10–15 minutes of walking or other aerobic activity)
Tuesday	Strength training (8–10 exercises; 1–2 sets of each; 10–15 repetitions with moderate loads)
Wednesday	Aerobics (10–15 minutes of walking or other aerobic activity)
Thursday	Strength training (8–10 exercises; 1–2 sets of each; 10–15 repetitions with moderate loads)
Friday	Aerobics (10–15 minutes of walking or other aerobic activity)
Saturday	Rest

Rate of progression: Each week, add 10 minutes to aerobic activity until you have reached 30–45 minutes of exercise. In the early stages of this routine, work out aerobically at an RPE of 11 or less; try to progress to an RPE of 12–14. On strength-training days, increase your weight loads by 5–10 pounds when you can comfortably accomplish 15–20 repetitions. Stay on this schedule for 4–8 weeks before advancing to the intermediate routine.

INTERMEDIATE EXERCISE ROUTINE	
Sunday	Optional aerobics (30–45 minutes)
Monday	Aerobics (30–45 minutes)
Tuesday	Strength training (8–10 exercises; 2–3 sets of each; 10–15 repetitions with moderate loads)
Wednesday	Aerobics (30–45 minutes)
Thursday	Strength training (8–10 exercises; 2–3 sets of each; 10–15 repetitions with moderate loads)
Friday	Aerobics (30–45 minutes)
Saturday	Strength training (8–10 exercises; 2 to 3 sets of each; 10–15 repetitions with moderate loads) Option: 45–60 minutes of aerobics instead of strength training

Rate of progression: Each week, add 10 minutes to aerobic activity until you have reached 45–60 minutes of exercise. Exercise aerobically at an RPE of 12–14. On strength-training days, increase your weight loads by 5–10 pounds when you can comfortably accomplish 15–20 repetitions. Stay on this schedule for 8–12 weeks before moving on to the advanced routine.

DIABETES AND SPORTS

Having diabetes need not stop you from being an athlete or competing in sports. Today, people with diabetes participate in practically every sport, from marathon running to football, and at all levels of competition. The key is learning how to carefully balance medication, diet, and exercise to avoid untoward blood sugar reactions when you train or compete.

ADVANCED EXERCISE ROUTINE

Sunday	Aerobics (45–60 minutes)
Monday	Aerobics (45–60 minutes)
Tuesday	Strength training (8–10 exercises; 3–5 sets of each; 10–15 repetitions with moderate loads)
Wednesday	Aerobics (45–60 minutes)
Thursday	Strength training (8–10 exercises; 3–5 sets of each; 10–15 repetitions with moderate loads)
Friday	Aerobics (45–60 minutes)
Saturday	Strength training (8–10 exercises; 3–5 sets of each; 10–15 repetitions with moderate loads) Option: Perform 45–60 minutes of aerobics instead of strength training

Rate of progression: Each week, add 10 minutes to aerobic activity until you have reached 45–60 minutes of exercise. Exercise aerobically at an RPE of 12–14. On strength-training days, increase your weight loads by 5–10 pounds when you can comfortably accomplish 15–20 repetitions.

Children with diabetes can play sports too. If your child has diabetes, talk to your pediatrician about any precautions that should be taken. In addition, find other parents of diabetic children and discuss with them which sports their children play. You will also find information about diabetes and sports in the resources section at the end of this book.

STICKING TO YOUR ROUTINE

One of the most challenging aspects of exercise is sticking to it. If you want to control your diabetes—and in doing so, look better, feel better, live better—you must get motivated and stay that way. Here are some suggestions.

Engage in Exercise You Enjoy

To make exercise a part of your life, it has to be fun—something you look forward to. But what if you're easily bored? Simply select several alternative fun activities such as a sport or recreation that will help you stay active.

Make Sure Exercise Is Convenient

Accessibility to pools, gyms, or other special facilities influences your decision to participate in certain activities. Ask yourself: Is the exercise readily available and affordable, scheduled at convenient times, easy to get to, or is it available only during certain seasons? Studies show that one of the major reasons people drop out of exercise programs is inconvenience. It's easier to stick to your routine when exercise is convenient and accessible.

Establish a Regular Schedule

In advance, schedule your exercise sessions on your calendar and then stick to them. A regular schedule makes all diabetes regimen adjustments easier to follow, improving glucose control all the more.

Exercise with a Friend

Exercising with a friend can motivate and encourage you, especially when you're tempted to skip a workout. For safety's sake too, a workout partner can help if you experience hypoglycemia or other problems during your exercise session.

Reward Yourself

If you've been faithful to your exercise routine and achieved any goals, reward yourself. Your reward should be a true treat, something you don't often do for yourself. Choose rewards that make you feel physically attractive or emotionally uplifted, or are just plain fun. Some examples: a massage, pampering at a day spa, new exercise shoes, a weekend getaway, a new outfit, or a donation to your favorite charity.

Your reward shouldn't tempt you to backslide. For instance, if you've just lost several pounds, don't reward yourself with a box of candy. Or if you've worked out faithfully for three weeks, don't take time off from exercise.

Keep a Long-Term Perspective

For people with diabetes, exercise is a vital therapeutic tool that, along with diet and medical care, is necessary for controlling and managing the disease. That being so, exercise as if your life depended on it, because in many cases, it does.

• • •

WHAT THE EXPERTS ADVISE:
Top-Ten Strategies for Exercise
Sheri Colberg, Ph.D.

Sheri Colberg, Ph.D., is the author of *The Diabetic Athlete*, which gives eighty-six sport-specific recommendations for regimen changes and other useful information about exercise

EXERCISE SELECTION

COMPLICATIONS	ACCEPTABLE EXERCISES*	DISCOURAGED EXERCISES
Heart disease	• Walking • Low-intensity activites	• High-intensity or strenuous exercises
Impaired circulation	• Walking • Swimming • Aquatic exercise • Stationary cycling • Non-weight-bearing activity	• Weight-bearing activities
Retinopathy	• Swimming • Walking • Low-impact (nonstraining, nonjarring) aerobics • Stationary cycling	• Strength training • Jogging • High-impact aerobics • Head-down activities • Racquet sports • Boxing • Heavy competitive sports
Nephropathy	• Low- to moderate-intensity activities	• Running • Aerobic dancing • Strength training • High-intensity or strenuous exercise

and guidelines for diabetes. She is an assistant professor of exercise science at Old Dominion University in Norfolk, Virginia, and is currently conducting research funded by the American Diabetes Association. Here are her top-ten exercise strategies for controlling diabetes during exercise.

1. Cardiovascular exercise (aerobic activity) results in the greatest improvements in your endurance capacity. However, resistance training is also an important means to increase lean

EXERCISE SELECTION (cont'd)		
COMPLICATIONS	**ACCEPTABLE EXERCISES***	**DISCOURAGED EXERCISES**
Neuropathy (distal or focal)	• Swimming • Bicycling • Rowing • Chair exercises • Arm exercises • Any non-weight-bearing exercise	• Treadmill • Prolonged walking or jogging • Step exercises (including stair-climbing machines and bench-stepping classes)
Neuropathy (autonomic)	• Low-intensity, indoor exercise, only with physician approval	• High-intensity or strenuous exercise • Outdoor exercise

*"Acceptable exercises" have been deemed safe to perform by your physician. Anyone with diabetes complications should obtain physician approval before beginning an exercise program. If you have complications, ask your physician about participating in a medically supervised exercise program.

Source: Adapted from American Diabetes Association. 2000. Diabetes mellitus and exercise. Position statement; American College of Sports Medicine. 2000. American College of Sports Medicine Position stand: Exercise and type 2 diabetes. *Medicine and Science in Sports and Exercise* 32: 1345–60.

body mass and improve your body's sensitivity to insulin. Include both forms of exercise during the week.

2. Your exercise intensity should reflect the goals of your training. If your primary goal is weight loss, doing an activity at a lower intensity for a longer period of time is usually a good choice. Also, you are less likely to drop out of your exercise program if your initial exercise intensity is not too hard. Start out easy, especially if you have been inactive, and then increase your exercise intensity as you feel ready.

3. An easy, subjective way to monitor your exercise intensity is using the rating of perceived exertion scale (see page 172). Your exercise should feel "somewhat hard" to "hard" to be effective for cardiovascular training. Working out at a

lower intensity still burns calories, but it may not have as great a training effect. Use the "talk test" as well: If you cannot comfortably talk during an activity, then you are exercising at a level that is too hard.

4. The recommended duration and frequency of exercise is twenty to sixty minutes done continuously at least three to five days per week. However, doing any exercise can help you control your blood sugar levels, even if it is shorter in duration or discontinuous. Add exercise throughout your day by taking the stairs instead of the elevator and walking as much as possible. It all adds up!

5. Incorporate regular stretching into your exercise routine. Joint mobility and flexibility can become limited with aging, and the effects of higher than normal blood sugar over time can worsen this problem. Stretch the major areas of your body that you are exercising for five to ten minutes before or after exercise, or both before and after.

6. Intense exercise (like sprinting or heavy weight training) can cause a large increase in your blood sugar due to your body's exaggerated release of glucose-raising hormones. Expect your blood sugar to be elevated for at least an hour or so following such activities.

7. Even if your blood sugar normally drops during exercise, you may find that several weeks of consistent training cause it to drop less than before. Thus, you may need to make changes in food or insulin (if taken) after training when doing the same exercise.

8. Carbohydrate is the most important energy source for your body during exercise. Since you are using more blood sugar as well, watch for any signs and symptoms of low blood sugar. If it starts to drop too low during an activity, you

should consume a rapidly absorbed carbohydrate food such as regular soda, juice, sport drink, hard candy (not chocolate), raisins, bread, or low-fat crackers.

9. If your blood sugar is elevated before exercise, you may not need to take any supplemental carbohydrate for a normal length activity. If starting in a normal blood sugar range, you may need to supplement with 10–30 grams of carbohydrate per hour, depending on your response. Your response will vary with the sport or activity. Test your blood sugar using your meter before, sometimes during, and after all activities to determine your individual response.

10. If you use supplemental insulin, you may need to dose with less before an activity, especially if it will be prolonged. Again, test your blood sugar to see your response before changing your insulin doses, and take extra carbohydrate as needed to prevent low blood sugar.

STEP FIVE

Take Medicine if Your Doctor Prescribes It

You can control your blood sugar swings by taking diabetes medicine prescribed by your doctor. These medicines include self-administered insulin (which is your lifeguard if you have type 1 diabetes) and any number of oral diabetes agents, which are sometimes prescribed for type 2 diabetes. In certain cases, you may also have to use insulin if you have type 2 diabetes.

Keep in mind that medications for type 2 diabetes are an adjunct to—not a replacement for—a nutritious diet and regular exercise program. Generally, your doctor will prescribe insulin and/or oral diabetes medications in type 2 diabetes only as a last resort, after you've made an honest stab at diet, exercise, and other healthy lifestyle practices. Even then, you might want to redouble your diet and exercise efforts, because they can reduce, or even eliminate, your need to take medicine. Luckily, oral diabetes drugs are a temporary fix in most cases, but they are still a monumentally important tool you can use to control your diabetes.

If your doctor does prescribe medicine, it's important to understand the medication you're taking, as well as when to take it, what side effects it may have, and how it works to keep your diabetes under control. Thus, in this step, you'll learn about:

- Insulin and how to use it
- The six classes of oral diabetes medicines and which ones may be right for you
- Oral combination therapy: why taking several of these medications may be necessary to normalize your blood sugar
- The importance of taking a low-dose aspirin every day to cut your risk of the number-one cause of death among diabetics—heart attack

INSULIN

You've probably wondered why insulin doesn't yet come in an easy-to-take pill. Insulin is a protein. Formulated as a pill, it would be broken down in your stomach, never get to your bloodstream, and be rendered useless. This is why you have to inject insulin.

No one likes shots. But it might help you to know that millions of people just like you take these injections every day without thinking much about it. How do they do it? Over time, they've gotten used to the shots and have come to appreciate the fact that insulin is making them feel better—and keeping them alive.

So if your doctor says you must take supplemental insulin, talk to other people with diabetes who use it. Chances are, you'll find that it doesn't slow them down or compromise their quality of life, but in fact gives them the control they need to do what they want. And the same will be true for you.

To start with, let's talk about insulin and answer some of the basic questions that are probably on your mind.

How Do I Give Myself Insulin Injections?

Injecting insulin doesn't always involve needles, although that's the way most insulin is delivered. Here's an explanation of the various ways to deliver insulin into your body, some of them needle-less.

Syringe. This consists of a needle, barrel, and plunger. The size of the syringe is matched to the strength of your insulin and to the dose you take. Your diabetes health care team will teach you how to use the syringe, including proper disposal.

Insulin injections are not as painful as you might imagine, for a couple of reasons. First, insulin is injected *subcutaneously*, which means "just under the skin." This area of the skin is made up of mostly fatty tissue, with very few nerve endings so you hardly feel the shot at all. Second, the needles are quite tiny, and some are coated with a special lubricant that eases them into the skin.

The syringe, lancet, and any other material that touches human blood are considered medical waste and should be placed in special containers with tight-fitting covers for disposal. Check with your doctor, pharmacist, and local health department to find out how to properly dispose of medical waste in your community.

Insulin pump. Worn on your body, this device releases a small, measured, and constant dose of insulin through a plastic tube. This delivery method most closely imitates your body's normal release of insulin and is termed a *basal dose*.

You can also pump extra insulin when you need it, such as before meals. This type of dose is called a *bolus dose*. If you use a pump, you must test your blood glucose levels at least four times a day and learn how to adjust insulin, diet, and exercise in response to the test results.

Generally, of your total daily insulin, about half should come from bolus doses, the other half from basal doses. Certain factors may change the basal dose you require, however. These include exercise, weight gain or loss of 5 to 10 percent of your body weight, increasing or decreasing blood glucose levels during your menstrual period, illness, and taking other medications. Your health care team will help you determine and set the appropriate adjustments.

There are a number of advantages to insulin pump therapy, for both type 1 and type 2 diabetes. Research shows that you may be able to achieve tighter glucose control using pump therapy and need less insulin. With pump therapy, you don't always have to carry around insulin vials and syringes.

Automatic injector. This device painlessly inserts a needle into your skin and releases the insulin. An automatic injector is advantageous if you have trouble holding a syringe or just can't bring yourself to give yourself a shot.

A jet injector is a needle-free device but works like a liquid needle, shooting insulin into your skin very rapidly with pressure rather than with a puncture. If you're afraid of needles, a jet injector is a good alternative. However, it can be costly and has to be disassembled every two weeks for sterilization.

Pen injector. This resembles a writing pen but has a disposable needle instead of a writing tip and an insulin cartridge instead of an ink cartridge. Each cartridge holds 150 units of insulin, and you can set the injector for the dose you need. Simply stick the needle in your skin and give yourself a shot of insulin.

Infuser. This is a special catheter needle, which can be inserted into your abdomen or other site to deliver insulin to the bloodstream. The needle can stay at the injection site for two or three days. With infusers, however, there is a greater risk of infection, so you must pay strict attention to sterile techniques.

Inhaled insulin. Diabetes researchers are working on new, less invasive ways to get insulin into your body. One of the most promising methods is inhaled insulin. This involves the use of a portable inhaler for insulin, similar to the device used by people with asthma. A study in a recent issue of the medical journal *Lancet* reported that people with type 1 diabetes who inhaled insulin kept their blood glucose levels as stable as those who injected it.

With inhaled insulin, the hormone is converted into a powder, which is placed into a device that aerosolizes it for absorption by the lungs. Researchers feel that the inhaler may benefit people with type 2 diabetes, as well. They caution, though, that more research is needed. So stay tuned—inhaled insulin could become the delivery system of choice in the future.

Liquid insulin. Another promising noninvasive delivery system for insulin is liquid insulin, now being tested in clinical trials. This form of insulin is swirled around in your mouth and then absorbed into the bloodstream. If it becomes available, liquid insulin will be prescribed for type 1 and type 2 diabetes.

Injection aids. If you have visual impairments, check out some of the special devices designed to make injections easier for you. These include needle guides, syringe magnifiers, and nonvisual measurement tools. Your diabetes health care team can provide information on products for people with visual impairments.

There are countless products available to make giving an injection seem effortless. The best source of information on insulin delivery is in the magazine *Diabetes Forecast*, which publishes an annual Buyer's Guide. You can also access the Buyer's Guide on-line at: www.diabetes.org/diabetesforecast.

Where Should I Inject Insulin?

The injection site has a lot to do with blood glucose control. This is because the rate at which insulin arrives in the blood is affected by the place on your body where you inject the insulin. For example, insulin works fastest when injected in the abdomen. By contrast, it enters the blood more slowly if injected into the upper arms, thighs, or buttocks.

For best results, inject insulin in the same general area. That way, you know that the insulin will reach its destination—the blood—with about the same speed with each injection. This gives you tighter glucose control and fewer blood sugar fluctuations. However, don't inject in the same exact spot every time, but move around the same general area. Injecting in the same spot every day can cause hard lumps or fat deposits to form. The *American Diabetes Association Complete Guide to Diabetes* advises that you make each shot a finger-length away from your last injection.

In addition, diabetes experts recommend that if you take several injections a day, you choose one body part per shot: the buttocks for morning shots, the abdomen for lunch shots, and the thigh for your evening shots, for example. Never inject in the two-inch area around your navel; its tough tissue causes wildly variable absorption rates of insulin. Ask your doctor or diabetes educator how best to rotate your injection sites.

How Often Should I Give Myself Insulin Injections?

Insulin plans employ one or two types of insulin and are designed to imitate the insulin secretion of a normal pancreas. Your physician will give you instructions on the number of shots you may need each day and will help you establish a personal insulin plan that fits your diet and lifestyle. Your insulin plan may

> ### HOW TO STORE INSULIN
>
> - Store the insulin you're using at room temperature, or warm the bottles between your hands before filling the syringe.
>
> - Store unopened bottles of insulin in your refrigerator. (Don't inject cold insulin, however, because it makes the shot more painful.)
>
> - Do not store insulin at temperatures under 36° Fahrenheit or over 86° Fahrenheit because insulin is destroyed at very high or very low temperatures. Never freeze your insulin or place it in direct sunlight.
>
> - Don't store open bottles of insulin at room temperature for more than a month, or they could become contaminated or lose their potency.
>
> - On the label, record the date you first opened the bottle.
>
> - Discard opened bottles you've used for a month.
>
> - Always check the expiration date before using insulin.
>
> - If your insulin ever looks unusual, don't use it. Return it to the pharmacy for an exchange or refund. Regular or lispro insulin should be clear, with no floating particles, color, or cloudiness. Intermediate-acting insulin should look cloudy, but without floating pieces or crystals.
>
> - Keep insulin out of the reach of children.

include one shot, two shots, three shots, or multiple shots a day and will be tailored to your individual needs.

ORAL DIABETES MEDICATIONS

Oral diabetes medications can help you live a near-normal life, plus help you stay complication-free. There are many medications available, so it's important to understand what your options are.

What follows is information on the six classes of oral medications available if you have type 2 diabetes. Be sure to read the section on aspirin too, to learn about its heart-protecting role in diabetes.

Sulfonylureas (sul-FON-ill-you-REE-ahs)

How do these drugs work? Used to treat type 2 diabetes for more than fifty years, sulfonylureas reduce blood glucose by stimulating your pancreas to produce more insulin.

There are many different types of sulfonylureas, and all have similar effects on blood glucose. Among the major sulfonylureas are Amaryl (glimepiride); Diabinese (chlorpropamide); Glucotrol and Glucotrol XL (glipizide); Diabeta, Glynase, and Micronase (glyburide); and Orinase (tolbutamide).

When should you take this medication? These drugs are generally taken one to two times a day, before meals. Your doctor may adjust your dosage up or down, based on your individual needs.

What are the potential side effects? Most of these agents are broken down by your liver and excreted by your kidneys. Thus, if you have liver or kidney problems, your doctor may advise against taking some sulfonylureas because your body will be unable to eliminate them properly.

These drugs may cause your blood glucose to dip too low (under 70 mg/dl), resulting in hypoglycemia. This can happen if you skip meals or consume too much alcohol.

Another potential side effect is weight gain. Also, if you are allergic to sulfa drugs, you should be careful about taking sulfonylureas.

Sulfonylureas should not be taken if you are suffering from diabetic ketoacidosis, a life-threatening medical emergency caused by insufficient insulin.

Nor should they be taken if you are pregnant or breast-feeding. One exception to this is Glucotrol. However, it should be taken only on the advice of your physician. Usually, Glucotrol is discontinued one month prior to the expected delivery date. Your doctor may advise you to discontinue Glucotrol while nursing.

The box on page 196 compares the major sulfonylureas.

Biguanides (by-GWAN-ides)

How do these drugs work? Used for decades in Europe, this class of medications came on the U.S. market in 1995. At present, there is only one biguanide available for use in the United States: Glucophage (metformin HCL tablets). Glucophage XR is the extended release version. Both versions have the same active ingredient.

Glucophage works differently from the sulfonylureas in that it does not increase insulin secretion from your pancreas. Instead it controls blood glucose by:

- Helping your body respond better to the insulin it makes naturally. This promotes the burning of sugar.
- Decreasing the amount of glucose made by your liver.
- Decreasing the amount of glucose absorbed by your intestines.

A benefit of using Glucophage is that, when taken alone, it rarely causes hypoglycemia or weight gain. However, when taken with a sulfonylurea or insulin, there is a greater chance of both conditions.

When should you take this medication? Glucophage is generally taken twice a day, with morning and evening meals. Your doctor will tailor your dosage to your individual needs. Glucophage XR is taken once a day.

What are the potential side effects? Common side effects

| SULFONYLUREAS ||||
BRAND NAME	**GENERIC NAME**	**DOSAGE**	**IMPORTANT ISSUES**
Amaryl	glimepiride	Once a day, usually with breakfast or the first main meal	Often prescribed with the insulin-boosting drug Glucophage
Diabinese	chloropropamide	Once a day, usually with breakfast	If you have a heart condition, discuss with your doctor the advisability of taking this medication
DiaBeta Glynase Micronase	glyburide	Once a day, usually with breakfast or the first main meal	Often prescribed with the insulin-boosting drug Glucophage
Glucotrol Glucotrol XL	glipizide	Once a day, 30 minutes before a meal (Glucotrol). Higher dosages are taken in two equal doses before meals. Glucotrol XL should be taken with breakfast.	Glucotrol XL tablets should be taken whole, not chewed, crushed, or divided. You may notice a tablet in your stool. This is only the empty shell that has been eliminated.
Orinase	tolbutamide	Generally taken once a day, 30 minutes before a meal.	Makes you susceptible to hypoglycemia if you have kidney or liver problems; lack enough adrenal or pituitary hormones; are elderly; are malnourished; overdo exercise or alcohol; or take more than one glucose-lowering drug

Source: Adapted from *The PDR Family Guide to Prescription Drugs.*

include diarrhea, nausea, and upset stomach. These generally go away the longer you are on the medication. Taking Glucophage with meals helps reduce these side effects.

A rare side effect of taking Glucophage is a serious and potentially fatal condition called *lactic acidosis*, which is a buildup of lactic acid in the blood. It occurs in people whose liver or kidneys are not working properly. Lactic acidosis is a medical emergency that requires treatment in a hospital. Symptoms of lactic acidosis may include weakness, tiredness, feelings of cold, dizziness, increasing sleepiness, unusual muscle pain, slow or irregular heartbeat, trouble breathing, or unexpected or unusual stomach discomfort.

According to *The PDR Family Guide to Prescription Drugs*, you should not take Glucophage if you:

- Have ever had an allergic reaction to this medication
- Suffer from congestive heart failure, a condition that increases your risk of developing lactic acidosis
- Suffer from ketoacidosis
- Are scheduled for an X-ray procedure that uses an injectable contrast agent (radioactive iodine). Do not take Glucophage for two days before and after having this procedure.
- Are going to have major surgery
- Have kidney or liver problems, or have developed serious conditions such as a severe infection, heart attack, or stroke
- Are seriously dehydrated
- Are pregnant or breast-feeding

Alpha-Glucosidase Inhibitors (al-fa-GLU-co-side-ase)

How do these drugs work? Alpha-glucosidase inhibitors reduce blood glucose levels by blocking the enzymes that digest starch in the intestines. Thus, following a meal, the absorption of sugar into the blood is delayed, and sudden upward surges of glucose are prevented. Precose (acarbose) and Glyset (miglitol) are the two drugs approved in this class.

Precose may be taken alone or together with certain other oral diabetes medications such as Diabinese, Micronase, Glucophage, and insulin. Glyset may be taken alone too, or in conjunction with a sulfonylurea to enhance glucose control.

When should you take these medications? Generally, these drugs are taken three times a day with the first bite of each main meal. Individual doses vary, and your doctor will adjust yours according to your response to the drug. While taking Precose, you will have blood tests every three months to see how your liver is reacting to the medication.

If you are taking either of these drugs with other diabetes medications, your blood sugar could dip too low. To counter this reaction, have on hand a source of glucose (such as glucose tablets) in case you experience mild to moderate hypoglycemia. Table sugar won't work because Precose and Glyset block its absorption.

What are the potential side effects? According to *The PDR Family Guide to Prescription Drugs*, common side effects associated with Precose are abdominal pain, diarrhea, and gas.

Similarly, common side effects of Glyset include gas, soft stools, diarrhea, or abdominal discomfort. These usually diminish with time.

You should not take Precose or Glyset if you:

- Suffer from ketoacidosis
- Have cirrhosis of the liver
- Have inflammatory bowel disease, ulcers in your colon, or any intestinal obstruction or chronic intestinal disease
- Are pregnant or breast-feeding

Thiazolidinediones (thigh-uh-ZO-la-deen-DYE-owns)

How do these drugs work? Thiazolidinediones are a class of medications that reduce insulin resistance. They help make cells more sensitive to your body's own insulin, rather than increase its insulin output. Thiazolidinediones also decrease sugar production in your body. Both actions help control hyperglycemia.

Currently, there are two thiazolidinediones on the market: Avandia (rosiglitazone maleate) and Actos (pioglitazone hydrocloride). Approved by the FDA in 1999, Actos is the newer of the two drugs.

Avandia is used alone or in conjunction with Glucophage. Actos is used alone or in combination with insulin injections or other oral diabetes drugs such as Diabeta, Micronase, Glucotrol, or Glucophage.

When should you take this medication? Avandia is taken once a day in the morning, or divided in half and taken in the morning and evening, with or without food. Actos is taken once a day, with or without meals.

What are the potential side effects? According to *The PDR Family Guide to Prescription Drugs*, common side effects with Avandia include back pain, fatigue, headache, high blood sugar, respiratory tract infections, sinus inflammation, and swelling. You should not take Avandia if you have liver disease. Before prescribing this drug, your physician will order tests to make sure your liver function is normal. Your liver will be rechecked every two months for the first year and periodically thereafter. Symptoms of liver damage include jaundice, nausea, vomiting, abdominal pain, fatigue, loss of appetite, and dark urine. If you notice any of these symptoms, notify your doctor right away.

According to *The PDR Family Guide to Prescription Drugs*, common side effects with Actos are headache, muscle aches, respiratory tract infection, sinus inflammation, sore throat, swelling, and tooth problems. With Actos, the FDA and manufacturer recommend having a liver test prior to taking the drug, every two months during the first year of therapy, and periodically thereafter. Report to your physician any symptoms that suggest liver disease.

In addition, you should not take Actos if you have heart problems, because the drug can cause swelling and fluid retention, which can aggravate heart disease. Swelling is more likely when Actos is combined with insulin.

Neither of these drugs should be taken if you are pregnant or nursing.

Meglitinides (meh-GLIT-in-ides)

How do these drugs work? This class of medications help the pancreas secrete more insulin, thus lowering blood glucose levels. Currently, Prandin (repaglinide) is the only agent of this class on the market.

Prandin may be prescribed alone, or in combination with Glucophage. If diet, exercise, and combination therapy fail to reduce your blood glucose, your physician may have to start you on insulin.

When should you take this medication? Prandin is taken two, three, or four times a day, usually about fifteen minutes before each meal.

What are the potential side effects? According to *The PDR Family Guide to Prescription Drugs*, common side effects include back pain, bronchitis, chest pain, constipation, diarrhea, headache, indigestion, joint pain, low blood sugar, nasal inflammation, nausea, sinus inflammation, skin tingling, upper respiratory tract infection, urinary tract infection, and vomiting. You should not take Prandin if you:

- Have type 1 diabetes
- Have ketoacidosis
- Have an allergic reaction to the drug
- Are pregnant (the effects of Prandin during pregnancy have not been well studied) or breast-feeding (it is not known whether the drug appears in breast milk)

D-Phenylalanine Derivatives (dee-fee-nil-AL-luh-neen)

How do these drugs work? The first in this new class of oral agents is Starlix (nateglinide), derived from the amino acid phenylalanine. The drug works by mimicking your body's own insulin patterns. Basically, it acts on the beta cells of the pancreas to stimulate rapid insulin secretion and reduce the surge in blood glucose after you eat a meal. It thus controls mealtime elevations in glucose. Once glucose levels are restored to normal, Starlix stops working.

Starlix can be taken alone, but it is also approved for use in combination with Glucophage. Research indicates that combination therapy is highly effective in achieving tighter glucose control.

When should you take this medication? One dose is taken three times a day, with each major meal. The drug comes in different dosages, and your doctor will determine which amount is right for you.

What are the potential side effects? The only side effects that have been reported thus far in clinical studies of Starlix are low blood sugar and a slight increase in body weight. Starlix should not be taken if you:

- Have type 1 diabetes
- Have ketoacidosis
- Are pregnant or nursing

ORAL COMBINATION THERAPY

If you're taking the maximum recommended dosage of an oral diabetes drug and still can't achieve good glucose control, your doctor may advise oral combination therapy. This may involve multiple pills (some of these combinations were described briefly in the drug descriptions), a single pill, or a combination of one or more oral diabetes medications and insulin.

Various combinations of oral medications are used to help achieve tighter glucose control. For example, a sulfonylurea (other than glyburide) may be prescribed along with Glucophage. In some cases, doctors may prescribe up to three drugs taken together. If your doctor prescribes multiple pills to treat your diabetes, be sure to take the medicine exactly as prescribed.

In combination, the drugs metformin and glyburide are often prescribed to treat type 2 diabetes. This combination of drugs is now available in a convenient single tablet in a glucose-lowering medicine called Glucovance. In studies, it has been found to be more effective in lowering blood sugar than either metformin or glyburide alone.

Glucovance is usually taken once or twice daily with meals. The side effects are similar to those you may experience with either metformin or glyburide: diarrhea, nausea, stomach upset, hypoglycemia, and rarely, lactic acidosis. According to the manufacturer, you should not take Glucovance if you:

- Have kidney problems
- Are eighty or older (unless you have your kidneys tested first)
- Are taking medication for heart failure
- Are seriously dehydrated

- Have a severe infection
- Have a history of liver disease
- Drink alcohol excessively

If oral combination therapy does not produce adequate glucose control, your physician may prescribe insulin, to be used along with your oral medications. The point of this approach is to try to make insulin work better.

Combinations usually include insulin with metformin, insulin with a sulfonylurea drug, or insulin with a thiazolidinedione. If used in combination with an oral agent, insulin is given once or twice a day. Follow your physician's advice to the letter when using insulin with oral diabetes medications.

ASPIRIN THERAPY IN TYPE 1 AND TYPE 2 DIABETES

A startling statistic: 98 percent of all people with diabetes are at risk of cardiovascular disease.

Happily, there's an incredibly easy way to drive down your risk, one that most people with diabetes should be doing but aren't: Take an aspirin a day. A study carried out by the Centers for Disease Control and Prevention (CDC) in Atlanta found that among those 98 percent at-risk people, only 20 percent were taking aspirin at least fifteen times a month.

Additional research shows that if you have diabetes, you can cut your risk of a heart attack by 60 percent as soon as you start taking aspirin. What's more, aspirin reduces the risk in both men and women, and in both those with type 1 and type 2 diabetes.

Why?

Aspirin is an *antiplatelet drug*. That means it prevents platelets—

tiny clotting substances in blood—from abnormally clumping together in a process called *platelet aggregation*. Platelet aggregation triggers the formation of dangerous blood clots called thrombi (singular, thrombus). A heart attack occurs when a thrombus obstructs a blood vessel supplying oxygen and nutrients to the heart muscle.

The American Diabetes Association now recommends that people with diabetes take an aspirin a day if they:

- Have cardiovascular disease
- Smoke
- Have high blood pressure
- Have cholesterol problems
- Have protein in the urine
- Are overweight
- Have a close family member (parent or sibling) who had a heart attack or stroke before the age of fifty

The recommended dosage is a daily baby aspirin, which contains 81 milligrams of aspirin, or one adult-strength 325-milligram aspirin daily.

Not everyone should use aspirin, however. Do not take aspirin if you're allergic to it, have a stomach ulcer, or suffer from active liver disease. If you are taking anticlotting drugs, aspirin may increase with their action. Consult your doctor about whether you are a candidate for aspirin therapy.

WHAT THE EXPERTS ADVISE:
Top-Ten Strategies for Getting the Best
Possible Medical Care

Richard P. Huemer, M.D., and Mary Kay Michelis, M.D.

Richard P. Huemer, M.D., has practiced nutritional and orthomolecular medicine since 1975. Dr. Huemer serves on the Los Angeles County Task Force on Nutrition and the International Board of Advanced Longevity Medicine. He is the associate editor of *Clinical Practice of Alernative Medicine*, a longtime health columnist for *Let's Live Magazine*, and the author (with Jack Challem) of *Natural Health Guide to Beating the Supergerms*.

Mary Kay Michelis, M.D., is a board-certified ophthalmologist and pioneer and innovator in ophthalmic surgery. The first female surgeon in the United States to implant an intraocular lens, she spearheaded a legal fight against the FDA in 1976 that resulted in these lenses becoming available to all Americans. Dr. Michelis was among the first to adopt refractive surgery, which she learned in Russia when radial keratotomy was still in its formative stages.

Here are their tips for assuring that you get the best possible medical care.

1. Select a doctor who is both knowledgeable about diabetes and sensitive to your needs for information and personal guidance.

2. Educate yourself about nutrition and proper diet, and how insulin is used; attend diabetes education classes at your local medical center.

3. Inform yourself about community resources available to you, including allied health professionals for your diabetes care team.

4. Understand how your blood sugar monitor works and what the numbers mean; use the monitor regularly.

5. Know the side effects of drugs used for diabetes, and promptly report to your doctor any that occur.

6. Get regular checkups with your doctor and others, including eye specialists.

7. Know how your body responds to certain foods; select the balance among carbohydrate, protein, and fat that works best for your own body.

8. Exercise regularly and consistently.

9. Understand the role of special nutrients in your condition: vitamins C and E, alpha-lipoic acid, chromium, vanadium, zinc, magnesium, acetyl-L-carnitine, and herbs.

10. Remember: Avoiding hypoglycemia requires several small meals a day.

STEP SIX

Defeat Stress with Positive Living

Your life is not the same after being diagnosed with diabetes. But this doesn't mean your life is necessarily worse, only different. Depending on your perspective, your life may even be better—if you look on your diagnosis as a wake-up call to take better care of yourself through nutrition, exercise, and other positive lifestyle changes. Diabetes doesn't have to limit you!

The key here is to control your diabetes so that it doesn't control you—a process that involves shoring up your emotional health. Doing so undergirds your ability to live with diabetes, ultimately leading to consistent, successful self-management. You see, when you're emotionally strong and well adjusted, you can better manage diet, exercise, medication, and other vital self-care strategies.

As you move toward better control of your diabetes, it's important to recognize how your mental state can affect the disease and what to do about negative emotions that can block your progress and stand in the way of better health.

In this step, you'll find out how to:

- Manage stress
- Defeat depression
- Fight your fears and phobias
- Tap into the power of healing relationships
- Improve your health through spiritual comfort

MANAGING STRESS

You've had a spat with your spouse. Your bills are past due. A deadline is looming. Your computer crashed. You've blown a sales call. The items on your to-do list exceed your capacity to do them.

In short, you're stressed out.

And it shows up in your blood glucose numbers, which have set a new altitude record.

When under stress, your body instantly prepares you to run from or contend with the situation—a reaction known as the fight or flight response. Your glands churn out the stress hormones adrenaline and cortisol, while your liver dispatches a surge of stored glucose to energize your muscles for sudden physical action. By contrast, some people physiologically react to stress with a drop in blood sugar. Hyperglycemia or hypoglycemia can trigger further stress through worry about the consequences or the feelings of fatigue both conditions can bring on. Stress also increases the need for insulin because the demands of stress overpower your body's ability to secrete the hormone. What's more, research shows that job stress is associated with high, unhealthy glycohemoglobin (GHb) measurements.

Under normal conditions, these stress reactions protect us from danger, but if stress goes unresolved and becomes chronic, there's trouble. Stress may speed up the development of type 2 diabetes, for example, because the body stops responding normally to insulin. The beta cells may stop producing enough insulin. Chronically high levels of stress hormones can lead to artery damage, cholesterol buildup, and heart disease, plus weaken your immune system.

When stressed out, you're likely to toss your diabetes self-care routine out the window. Rather than watch your diet, you might self-medicate by overindulging on comfort foods or alcohol. Or you might forgo your exercise program and collapse on the couch instead. You don't feel like monitoring your glucose either or taking your medicine, so you don't.

By itself, having diabetes is stressful enough, physically and mentally. You worry about developing complications, experiencing a hypoglycemic reaction in public, monitoring glucose, getting discouraged or anxious over the numbers, or taking medicine throughout the day. The list goes on.

Naturally, all of these reactions and behaviors lead to a loss of control over your diabetes.

So what's a stressed-out body to do? Here are some suggestions.

Fortify yourself nutritionally. Stress steals away nutrients. Make sure you follow your meal-planning system and eat a variety of healthy foods daily. Equally important, take a daily multivitamin/mineral/antioxidant supplement as nutritional insurance.

Get moving. No matter what's going on, try to exercise. It's one of the most effective ways to dissipate physical and emotional stress because it speeds up the production of feel-good chemicals called endorphins. Exercise also relieves stress-induced muscular tension.

Learn effective coping skills. Mental health therapists say that there are various types of skills you can employ to deal with stressors. One is to try to identify the source of the stress; then fix it. Let's say you're in debt over your head. Fixing the problem may involve working with a financial counselor to set up a debt repayment plan and changing your personal spending behaviors to avoid debt in the future.

Another coping strategy is to change your reaction to a stressor. This works best when dealing with difficult people or intolerable situations over which you have no control. The next time you are faced with something you can't control, find the humor in the situation, or downplay the severity of the situation. Ask yourself: What is the worst thing that can happen? How likely is that to occur? How much difference will this situation make in my life a year from now? Am I likely to even remember it? This type of response puts a more positive spin on the situation.

Breathe. Breathing exercises can help you lower stress in an instant. Sit or lie down and take in very deep breaths, while relaxing your muscles. Breathe and relax for five to twenty minutes a session, at least once a day.

Get enough rest. If you're an emotional basket case right now, take it easy by getting more rest. Rest lets your body renew itself.

Seek professional help. Sometimes, resolving stress requires more serious measures—like seeing a counselor. A counselor won't solve your stress problems, but he or she may help you identify strategies to cope with it and ultimately resolve the underlying issues perpetuating the stress. If you ever have thoughts of suicide, see a qualified counselor right away.

It is vital to select a good counselor, with good credentials. He or she should be someone you admire and respect, a person with whom you can maintain a counseling relationship. Your counselor should show professionalism too, adhering to confidentiality and standards of ethics. Make sure your counselor works with you to establish therapy goals and tailors a counseling approach for your personal situation.

DEFEATING DEPRESSION

Everyone feels down in the dumps occasionally. But if feelings of sadness or despair persist, day in and day out, without letting up, you could be suffering from clinical depression, a very serious psychiatric illness that affects both mind and body, as well as your quality of life.

Clinical depression strikes 15 to 20 percent of people with diabetes, whether it's type 1 or type 2—a rate that is three times higher than that of the general population. What's more, depression is twice as common in women than in men.

No one has yet clarified exactly why depression is so prevalent among people with diabetes, but there are some research-supported clues. Studies strongly suggest that situational factors associated with diabetes—daily dietary monitoring, blood sugar testing, the demands of medication, hospitalizations, and the financial burdens of treatment—can all trigger a protracted episode of the blues. Dealing with diabetic complications such as loss of vision, impotence, heart disease, kidney failure, or other health problems can certainly bring on a sense of despair too.

The origins of clinical depression among people with diabetes may also lie in biochemical changes associated with the disease. When your blood sugar is too high (hyperglycemia), you experience low energy, fatigue, and sleeplessness—symptoms that make you feel depressed. Just the opposite of hyperglycemia is hypoglycemia (low blood sugar). It produces depressive symptoms too: fatigue, mood changes, lack of concentration, and feelings of pessimism. Also, glucose intolerance and insulin resistance may cause chemical changes in the brain that lead to depression.

How can you tell if you've just got the doldrums or are wrestling with full-blown clinical depression? The disorder manifests itself in the following symptoms:

- Low energy and fatigue
- Persistent sadness
- Anxiety and tension
- Insomnia
- Loss of interest in pleasurable activities, including sex
- Memory problems, forgetfulness, poor concentration
- Irritability and crankiness with little or no provocation
- Unhappiness
- Lack of self-esteem
- Appetite problems, either loss of appetite or overeating
- Mood swings
- Thoughts of suicide

If you have three or more of these symptoms and they persist for two weeks or longer, you should seek help right away. People with diabetes who suffer from depression tend to have poorly controlled blood glucose, which ultimately can cause serious diabetes complications. Depression can also lead to obesity, physical inactivity, and substance abuse—all of which will further compromise your health.

Fortunately, though, depression is the most treatable of all emotional problems, and there are treatment options your doctor can recommend. The two most effective types of treatment in use today are medication and psychotherapy, and many patients benefit from a combination of the two. In fact, research shows that most people with diabetes who undergo psychotherapy and take antidepressant medication can be cured of depression within six months. Also significant: Studies show that when depression lifts, blood glucose levels improve.

Antidepressants

The major antidepressants used to treat diabetes include Prozac (fluoxetine), Paxil (paroxetine), Zoloft (sertraline), Elavil (amitriptyline), and Pamelor (nortriptyline). The first three on the list are medically known as *selective serotonin reuptake inhibitors* (SSRIs). When you are depressed, there may be a short supply of neurotransmitters (chemical messengers) in your brain. This shortage blocks the transmission of messages between brain cells. Consequently, you feel down, sluggish, apathetic, and often hopeless. SSRIs act only on serotonin, a mood-regulating neurotransmitter. Serotonin levels are linked to feelings of calm and well-being. SSRIs lengthen the amount of time that concentrations of serotonin stay active in the brain, elevating your mood and making you feel better.

Elavil and Pamelor are tricyclic antidepressants (TCAs), which, like other antidepressants, work on brain chemicals. TCAs slow the rate at which certain neurotransmitters—serotonin, norepinephrine, and dopamine—reenter the brain. This action increases the concentration of the neurotransmitters throughout the rest of the central nervous system, alleviating feelings of depression.

Antidepressants are not without side effects—including hyperglycemia in some cases—and you should discuss these with your physician and pharmacist. Some alternative health care practitioners treat diabetes-related depression with an herb called Saint-John's-wort. It does not appear to affect blood sugar levels.

Counseling

A form of psychotherapy that is working mood-lifting wonders in clinically depressed patients with diabetes is *cognitive behavior therapy* (CBT). Developed by renowned psychiatrist Aaron Beck, CBT takes the view that depression stems from patterns of disordered thinking. It encourages you to change unrealistic and negative thinking and replace it with more accurate and useful thinking. CBT also emphasizes strategies to get you involved in good-for-you social and physical activities, plus teaches problem-solving skills for handling stressful situations. With CBT, you learn how to slip out of self-defeating thought patterns and think more positively and realistically about the world around you.

In a study conducted at Washington University in St. Louis, people with type 2 diabetes who were clinically depressed underwent CBT for ten weeks and were followed up six months later. By the end of ten weeks, depression had lifted in 85 percent of those who had had CBT. At the end of the six-month follow-up, 70 percent of the patients in CBT were still in remission from depression.

Other Secrets of Emotional Fitness

In addition to drug therapy and psychotherapy, other lifestyle changes can help you chase away the blues. These changes include many of the same strategies recommended for managing stress: nutrition, exercise, and adequate sleep.

Joining a diabetes support group to meet with other people

who share your problem can be an effective form of therapy, especially when combined with individual counseling. Topics typically discussed include strategies for diabetes control, family relationships, diabetes products, depression, and medication. Sharing with others helps address underlying problems contributing to depression and helps you see that you're not alone in your struggle.

Studies have been conducted on the benefit of support groups in controlling diabetes and alleviating depression, and the results are encouraging. In one study of people with type 1 or type 2 diabetes, those who participated in a diabetes education program followed by eighteen months of participation in a support group experienced less depression and stress, improved blood sugar control, and better quality of life than patients not in support groups.

Another study found that people with type 1 and type 2 diabetes who had little social support had significantly higher levels of glycated hemoglobin (11.8 percent on average) than those with strong support. There's a lot to be gained physically and emotionally by surrounding yourself with people who understand and share your situation.

An alternative to a traditional support group is an on-line support group, or moderated chat group, conducted via the Internet and sponsored by a health care organization. These are growing in popularity. Check with your local hospital or mental health center for information on Web sites in which such groups are active. Make sure the on-line support group is sponsored by a credible medical organization.

FIGHTING FEARS AND PHOBIAS

Perhaps you're preoccupied by the possibility of suffering complications of diabetes. Or you're worried you might have an insulin reaction while driving or out in public. Maybe you're afraid of needles, or petrified at the sight of blood.

Fear is an understandable reaction to any disease, and diabetes is no exception. But if the fear becomes so paralyzing that you won't leave your house, monitor your blood sugar, or give yourself an injection, you may be suffering from a phobia that will affect your health for the worse.

Basically, a phobia is the fear of a place, a situation, or an object. Phobias run the gamut from the simple, like the fear of insects, to the emotionally paralyzing, fear of being in public places, for example. There are hundreds of different kinds of phobias, and everyone has one or two.

A phobia is a concern only if it regularly interferes with and compromises your health and quality of life. A phobic person will go to great lengths to avoid the situation he or she fears, and that can be dangerous, particularly if it prevents compliance with diabetic self-care.

Phobias can be successfully overcome with a combination of medication, counseling, and gradual exposure to the fear-evoking situation. Medications commonly used to treat phobias include benzodiazepines and monoamine oxidase (MAO) inhibitors. Benzodiazepines are a class of drugs that include Valium (diazepam), Tranxene (clorazepate), Serax (oxazepam), Ativan (lorazepam), and Xanax (alprazolam). They produce their calming effect by interacting with a group of brain cells located in the limbic system, the area of your brain that controls emotions.

MAOs are antidepressants generally reserved for patients

with depression accompanied by symptoms of anxiety or phobias. The most commonly prescribed drugs in this group are Nardil (phenelzine sulfate) and Parnate (tranylcypromine). These drugs work by blocking monoamine oxidase, an enzyme that destroys serotonin and norepinephrine in the brain. Thus, by interfering with its action, MAO inhibitors help restore normal mood states. MAOs are up to 80 percent effective in treating phobias. Discuss with your physician the advisability of using such medications.

Phobias are also treated with psychotherapy to work through the problem. Part of this therapy may include *systematic desensitization,* in which you're gradually exposed to the thing you fear. With time, the object or situation will supposedly generate less fear the more you're exposed to it.

THE HEALING POWER OF LOVING, SUPPORTIVE RELATIONSHIPS

If your doctor could write a single prescription for good health, it would be, in a word, *love.* It's well known scientifically that the ability to love and be loved enhances the function of natural disease-fighting cells in your body and activates protective healing systems. When you feel loved, you're less likely to get sick. And if ill, your health will improve when you're surrounded by nurturing, caring people.

As with many chronic diseases, diabetes and its control are strongly influenced by the quality of relationships with family and friends. So say several studies that have looked into the association between social support and diabetes control.

In one study, researchers found that diabetic men living with supportive families, in which there was "low conflict" and less anxiety, had improved glucose control, lower glycated hemoglobin scores, and healthier cholesterol and triglycerides levels. By contrast, another study (involving adults with type 1 diabetes) revealed that those with nonsupportive family members were less likely to comply with their glucose testing, insulin, and nutritional therapies, plus had higher glycohemoglobin (GHb) scores.

Another study observed that women with gestational diabetes with strong social support were more successful at sticking to their diets and insulin therapy than women without such a network.

Numerous other research involving social support and diabetes shows that:

- Loving relationships with "significant others" influence your diabetes self-care program for the better.
- Supportive family members are instrumental in helping you adhere to insulin injections, glucose monitoring, and diet; close friends can provide needed emotional support.
- Social support contributes to emotional well-being and greater psychological adjustment. In one survey of people with diabetes, respondents stated that social support from family, friends, and support groups were major factors that helped them adjust to diabetes.

Clearly, it's important to make sure your relationships are short on conflict and long on understanding. But often that's challenging, particularly in some families. If your family situation is contentious, you may want to seek family therapy to help work through the conflict and move toward stronger support.

On a different note: Sometimes conflict stems from the understandable sadness, stress, anger, or anxiety experienced by family members after learning about your diagnosis. But according to a

University of Pittsburgh study, these negative emotions gradually fade, usually about one year after the diagnosis when the family returns to normal functioning and grows stronger.

The key in all of this is to avoid becoming lonely and isolated. Loneliness drives some people to unhealthy behaviors such as smoking, overeating, and substance abuse. Studies also show that loneliness can significantly increase the chances of various diseases, even premature death.

Seek out the companionship of others—people who stick close by to love, care, and listen when you need it most. The best way to have true friends is to be one. There are people who need your friendship and support as much as you need theirs.

SEEKING SPIRITUAL COMFORT

When African-American women with diabetes were asked in focus groups what influenced most positively the course of their disease, they responded with something that has been described as one of the greatest healers of all time: spiritual faith.

Their response would come as no surprise to the growing number of researchers who have discovered that having faith improves the outcome of disease, speeds recovery from illness, lowers blood pressure, enhances the immune system, prevents the likelihood of premature death, among other amazing benefits. Plus, there is a documented scientific link between faith and mental health. People who are religious or come from a religious family have a lower risk of suicide, mental health problems, drug abuse, alcoholism, and depression. Further, a string of scientific evidence suggests that spiritual well-being—defined as satisfaction with your life in relationship to God or a higher power and a perception of life as having meaning—is a valuable resource to help you cope in times of stress and illness. It also influences your emotional well-being.

What's more, regular attendance at church, synagogue, mosque, or other house of worship has a profound effect on your health. Researchers at Johns Hopkins University found that cardiovascular disease is much lower among people who have a lifetime of church attendance. Further, researchers at the University of Texas who analyzed surveys from twenty-one thousand American adults discovered that people who never attend church have almost twice the risk of death compared to those who attend more than once a week. And a Duke University study found higher levels of an immune-boosting substance called interleukin-6 in church-attending patients with diabetes, AIDS, Alzheimer's disease, osteoporosis, depression, and other illnesses.

Why such an impact?

Researchers believe that having faith gives you peace and hope, feelings that reduce stress, anxiety, and depression; motivates you to take better care of yourself (religiously committed people are less likely to pursue health-abusing behaviors such as drinking and smoking); and links you to a community of people who will love and support you—an atmosphere that is good for your body and soul.

Where diabetes is concerned, a study conducted at the University of Texas at Galveston produced some fascinating findings on the value of spiritual faith. The researchers surveyed ninety-four men and women who had either type 1 or type 2 diabetes and asked them various questions about their experiences with the disease, including adjustment to diabetes, management of the disease, and their use of spiritual resources. The researchers learned that those people with a high degree of spiritual well-being psychologically adjusted to and coped with the disease better than those without such faith. Also noteworthy: As spiritual well-being strengthened, problems related to living with diabetes decreased. So did feelings of uncertainty about the future.

POSITIVE LIVING

Controlling diabetes is a long-term process, with good days and not-so-good days. Sometimes, your blood glucose levels will hit their targets, and other days they'll be off. That's okay. Your goal should be to do as well as possible as often as you can, rather than obsess over the few times when your blood glucose is off.

Sometimes, people with diabetes fret over a few deviations and equate them with failure. Their internal dialogue becomes largely negative "self-talk." Suppose you say to yourself: "I'm a total failure because my glucose is out of control." There's no truth in such a statement. Surely you've had plenty of successes in your life, so there's no way you can be a "total failure." What's more, controlling or not controlling glucose isn't an accurate yardstick of your success or failure as a person.

A lot of the stuff we tell ourselves about ourselves is a distortion of the truth, or not truthful at all. Try to dissect your self-talk and decipher whether there's really any truth in it. Then replace the untruth with true, logical statements about yourself. Using the example above, you might tell yourself: "I'm not a failure. My commitment to controlling my diabetes is a sign of success. Every time I make even one healthy choice, I am succeeding."

If all you do is concentrate on the negative, you'll experience needless stress, anxiety, and depression. Keep in mind too that your goals will change over time, with your schedule, lifestyle, and overall health.

Some important advice in all of this is to adopt a just-for-today attitude. If you do, you'll find it much easier to stick to your diabetes self-care program. Successful behavior change takes small, daily steps. Focusing only on what you must do in a single day is a cinch compared to thinking about what you might have to do over a lifetime.

• • •

WHAT THE EXPERTS ADVISE:
Top-Ten Strategies for Emotional Well-Being
Judith Schwambach, Ph.D.

Mental health counselor, newspaper columnist, and author Judith Schwambach, Ph.D., is known as "Dr. Judith" to her clients, readers, and others. In addition to her office practice, she provides anonymous on-line counseling at her Web site: www.drjudith.com. Here are her top-ten tips for achieving emotional health if you have diabetes:

1. Buy an inexpensive notebook and chronicle your thoughts each day. Journaling is a great way to stay in touch with your emotions as you adjust to the impact of diabetes on your life. This provides a safe, consistent release for feelings that can otherwise pile up.

2. Join or start a diabetes support group and faithfully attend the meetings. This regular reminder that you are not alone in your battle is one of your best defenses against self-pity.

3. Keep a growing list of every good thing that is going on in your life. When you find yourself becoming discouraged about your diabetes, bring out your list and meditate briefly on each positive. In minutes, you'll begin to regain a healthy perspective.

4. Refuse to see yourself as a victim. Instead, learn everything you can about diabetes and take control. Knowledge is power. A thorough reading of this book is an excellent first step.

5. Make it manageable. Come up with half a dozen things that are worse than having diabetes, so the next time you start to feel overwhelmed, you can say, "At least I don't have _____."

6. Each day, take at least one Pleasure Break from thinking about diabetes, or any other problem. Lose yourself in something you truly enjoy. You'll come out of your break feeling refreshed and energized.

7. Carefully select an experienced person with diabetes to whom you can relate as a mentor. You need a knowledgeable, empathetic adviser you can turn to when you have questions or become discouraged.

8. Turnabout is fair play. Keep your eyes open for someone who has just been diagnosed with diabetes and let him or her know you are willing to help. When you're giving as well as receiving, you discover purpose in what you've endured.

9. Recognize the signs of clinical depression. If you cannot bounce back with the help of friends and family, see a qualified counselor and get professional help. The longer you permit yourself to remain depressed, the harder it is to dig out.

10. Don't hesitate to reach out to God. Every battle against disease has a spiritual component. A growing number of studies make it clear. People with strong faith cope better.

Glossary

advanced glycated end products (AGEs). Agents that are formed when glucose links up (or glycates) with substances in the blood. An excess of AGEs in the body can damage organs.

alpha-glucosidase inhibitors. Oral diabetes agents that reduce blood glucose levels by blocking the enzymes that digest starch in the intestines. Precose (acarbose) and Glyset (miglitol) are the two drugs approved in this class.

amino acids. Building blocks of protein necessary for growth and metabolism.

antioxidant. A special class of nutrients that fight free radicals, unstable molecules that damage healthy cells.

atherosclerosis. Narrowing of the arteries caused by deposits of cholesterol, fats, and other substances.

autoimmunity. A condition in which the immune system attacks the body's own cells. Type 1 diabetes is an autoimmune disease.

beta cells. Cells that produce insulin. Beta cells are located in the islets of Langerhans in the pancreas.

biguanides. Oral diabetes medications that lower glucose by promoting the burning of sugar, decreasing the amount of glucose produced by the liver, and decreasing the intestinal absorption of glucose. Glucophage is a biguanide.

blood glucose meter. A handheld device that tests and calculates blood glucose levels.

carbohydrate counting. A meal-planning system recommended for people who take supplemental insulin. This system estimates the number of carbohydrates in food and matches that amount to units of insulin.

carbohydrates. A food group that serves as a major energy source for the body. Derived mostly from sugar and starch, carbohydrate is broken down into glucose during digestion and is the main nutrient that elevates blood glucose levels.

cholesterol. A fatty substance found in some foods and manufactured by the body for many vital functions. Excess cholesterol and saturated fat can increase blood levels of cholesterol and can collect inside artery walls. This process contributes to heart disease.

creatinine. A substance in blood that is measured to detect the presence of kidney problems.

diabetes. A disease in which the body cannot produce enough insulin or cannot use insulin in a normal way. This leads to high levels of glucose in the blood.

diabetologist. A physician who specializes in the treatment of diabetes.

D-phenylalanine derivative. A new class of oral diabetes medications that mimics the body's own insulin patterns. There is currently one drug in this class: Starlix.

endocrinologist. A physician who specializes in treating diseases of the glands and also treats people with diabetes.

essential fatty acids (EFAs). Vitamin-like substances that have a protective effect on the body. They are called essential because the body cannot manufacture them. They must be obtained from food.

exchange list. A meal-planning system that includes seven basic food groups: starch, other carbohydrates, meat and meat substitutes, vegetable, fruit, milk, and fat.

fats. A food group that provides energy but is the most concentrated source of calories in the diet.

fatty acids. Components of either dietary fat or body fat.

fiber. The nondigestible portion of plants that can lower fat and glucose absorption and promote a healthy digestive system.

free radicals. Harmful molecules that destroy healthy cells by robbing them of oxygen; this robbery weakens the immune system.

fructose. A simple sugar found in fruit and fruit juices.

galactose. A simple sugar that is a part of lactose (milk sugar).

gestational diabetes. A form of diabetes that develops during pregnancy. Hormones secreted during pregnancy cause a rise in the mother's blood glucose, and the mother's body cannot produce enough insulin to handle the excess.

glucagon. A hormone produced by the pancreas that raises blood glucose levels. An injectable form is available by prescription and used to treat a severe insulin reaction.

glucose. Blood sugar. It acts as a fuel for the body.

glucose tolerance. The ability to transport blood glucose into cells for use by the body.

Glucovance. An oral diabetes medication formulated with a combination of metformin and glyburide. It is a blood sugar-lowering agent.

glycemic index of foods. A system of rating foods according to how fast they elevate blood glucose. Foods lower on the scale—low-glycemic-index foods—are sometimes recommended in nutritional therapy for diabetes.

glycogen. Stored carbohydrate in the muscles and liver.

glycohemoglobin (GHb) test. This test measures average blood sugar over a two- to three-month period. Glucose in the blood attaches itself to hemoglobin, a protein that carries oxygen in the blood. This glucose-hemoglobin substance, called glycated hemoglobin, stays in the blood for up to four months. In this test, the level of glycated hemoglobin indicates that average amount of glucose that was not metabolized for energy over a two- to three-month period. Also called glycated or glycosylated hemoglobin test.

glycosuria. Glucose in the urine.

high-density lipoprotein (HDL). A type of cholesterol in the blood that has a protective effect against the buildup of plaque in the arteries. So-called good cholesterol.

hyperglycemia. A condition in which blood glucose levels are too high, generally greater than 250 mg/dl.

hypoglycemia. A condition in which blood glucose levels fall too low, generally below 70 mg/dl.

immune system. A complex network of various types of cells and organs that work together to fight disease, from the common cold to deadly cancers.

impaired glucose tolerance (IGT). The inability of the body to properly break down and use glucose. IGT often precedes type 2 diabetes and is a risk factor for the disease. A glucose tolerance test can detect IGT.

impotence. Inability to have or sustain an erection of the penis. Often a result of nerve damage in diabetes.

insulin. A hormone that decreases blood glucose levels by moving glucose into cells to be used for fuel.

insulin pump. A device that delivers a steady release of insulin (basal dose) but can also deliver a large dose prior to meals (bolus dose).

insulin reaction. High blood sugar as a result of too much injected insulin for the amount of food or exercise.

insulin resistance. A condition in which the body does not respond to glucose properly, seen most commonly in type 2 diabetes. It is a major risk factor in type 2 diabetes.

intermediate-acting insulin. Insulin that reaches the bloodstream about two to four hours after it is injected, peaks four to twelve hours later, and continues to work for eighteen to twenty-four hours.

islet cells. Specialized cells in the pancreas that are arranged in clusters, or islets. There are four types of islet cells: alpha, beta, PP cells, and D1 cells. Insulin is released from beta cells.

ketoacidosis. A serious condition caused by the lack of insulin or an elevation in stress hormones. It produces high blood glucose levels and ketones in the urine. Ketoacidosis occurs most often in people with type 1 diabetes.

ketones. By-products of the breakdown of fat for fuel.

lactic acidosis. A rare but serious condition brought on by the buildup of lactic acid in the blood. Lactic acid is a waste product of glucose metabolism. Lactic acidosis can be fatal.

lactose. The simple sugar found in milk.

lancet. The fine needle used to prick skin for a blood glucose test.

long-acting insulin. Insulin that reaches the bloodstream six to ten hours after injection, peaks in fourteen to twenty-four hours, and continues to work for twenty to thirty-six hours. This form of insulin provides a near-continuous release of the hormone.

low-density lipoproteins (LDL). A type of cholesterol in the blood. High levels contribute to coronary heart disease. So-called bad cholesterol.

macrosomia. The condition of a baby at birth when the mother's gestational diabetes is not controlled. Also termed "fat baby."

macular edema. A swelling of the macula, an area near the center of the retina that is responsible for fine or reading vision. Macular edema is a common complication associated with diabetic retinopathy.

meglitinides. A class of medications that help the pancreas secrete more insulin, thus lowering blood glucose levels. Prandin (repaglinide) is a meglitinide.

metabolic rate. The speed at which the body burns calories.

metabolism. The physiological process that converts food to energy so that the body can function.

mg/dl (milligrams per deciliter). The unit of measure when describing blood glucose levels.

microalbuminuria. Abnormal amounts of protein in the urine.

minerals. Nutrients needed by the body for a wide range of enzymatic and metabolic functions.

monounsaturated fat. Fatty acids that lack two hydrogen atoms. Found in such foods as olive oil, olives, avocados, cashew nuts, and cold-water fish such as salmon, mackerel, halibut, and swordfish.

nephropathy. Kidney disease. A life-threatening complication of diabetes.

neuropathy. Nerve damage and a complication of diabetes.

obesity. An excessive and abnormal amount of weight, usually 20 percent or more above a person's ideal weight. Obesity is the chief risk factor for type 2 diabetes.

ophthalmologist. A physician who specializes in treating diseases of the eye.

oral diabetes agents. Medications taken by mouth that are designed to lower blood sugar. They are usually prescribed for people with type 2 diabetes and are not to be confused with insulin.

pancreas. A flask-shaped organ situated behind and just below the stomach. Its job is to secrete powerful digestive enzymes for the breakdown of food and to promote the production of insulin from beta cells in the pancreas.

periodontal disease. Infection and damage to the gums. Often a complication of diabetes.

podiatrist. A medical professional who specializes in treating the feet.

polyunsaturated fat. A fatty acid found in fish and in most vegetable oils.

protein. Food group necessary for growth and repair of body tissues.

rapid-acting insulin (lispro). Insulin that starts working within five minutes, peaks within sixty minutes, and continues to work for approximately three to four hours.

receptor. A physiological signal device located on the membrane of a cell. Receptors recognize substances such as hormones, nutrients, or drugs and allow access to the cell.

regular insulin. Insulin that reaches the bloodstream within thirty minutes after injection, peaks in about two to three hours after injection, and continues to work for about three to six hours. Also called short-acting insulin.

retina. The light-sensing part of the eye.

retinopathy. Damage to tiny blood vessels in the eye that can lead to vision problems. Retinopathy is a severe complication of diabetes.

saturated fat. A fatty acid that is solid at room temperature.

short-acting insulin. *See* **regular insulin.**

simple sugar. A type of carbohydrate that is constructed of either single or double molecules of glucose.

sorbitol. A breakdown product of excess glucose in the blood. An accumulation of sorbitol can cause tissue damage. (Sorbitol is also a sugar alcohol used to sweeten foods.)

stress hormones. Hormones released when the body is under stress. Stress hormones include cortisol, adrenaline, norepinephrine, and growth hormone.

sugar. A form of carbohydrate that supplies calories and can elevate blood glucose levels.

sulfonylureas. Oral diabetes medications that reduce blood glucose by stimulating the pancreas to produce more insulin.

syndrome X. A cluster of symptoms that set the stage for type 2 diabetes and heart disease. These symptoms include glucose intolerance, central obesity, elevated blood fats, and high blood pressure.

thiazolidinediones. A class of oral diabetes medications that reduce insulin resistance by making cells more sensitive to the body's own insulin. Actos and Avandia are members of this class of drugs.

triglycerides. Fats that circulate in the blood until they are deposited in fat cells.

type 1 diabetes. A form of diabetes that usually develops prior to age thirty but may occur at any age. It is caused by an immune system attack on the body's own beta cells. When these cells are destroyed, insulin can no longer be produced.

type 2 diabetes. A form of diabetes that typically occurs in people over age forty but can develop in younger people. With type 2 diabetes, the body does not use insulin properly.

unsaturated fat. Fat that is liquid at room temperature.

urine test. Test that measures substances in the urine, including ketones.

very-low-density lipoproteins (VLDL). A harmful type of cholesterol.

vitamins. Organic substances found in food that perform many vital functions in the body.

Resources

ORGANIZATIONS

For additional information, look to medical associations and organizations that help people with diabetes. These groups are among the best authorities for detailed and up-to-date information to help control your diabetes. Here are key organizations that can provide you with additional information on diabetes.

American Association of Diabetes Educators (AADE)
444 North Michigan Avenue
Suite 1240
Chicago, IL 60611
(312) 644-2233 or (800) 338-3633
www.aadenet.org

A professional organization representing more than ten thousand health professionals who provide diabetes education and care. Its Web site features a tool that helps you locate a diabetes educator in your community.

American Diabetes Association (ADA)
1660 Duke Street
Alexandria, VA 22314
(703) 549-1500 or (800) 232-3472
www.diabetes.org

Both a professional association and a private, nonprofit, voluntary organization with state and local affiliates and chapters. The ADA exists to serve people with diabetes and their families, as well as health professionals and scientists involved in diabetes-related activities. Its mission is "to prevent and cure diabetes and to improve the lives of all people affected by it." The ADA has a wealth of information available: monthly and quarterly magazines for patients, including *Diabetes Forecast*; professional journals for health care professionals; cookbooks, planning guides, and brochures for patients; and materials for health care professionals. The ADA's Web site is a highly useful source of easy-to-understand information on virtually every subject relating to diabetes.

To order American Diabetes Association books: Call 1-800-232-6733; Web site: store.diabetes.org.

To join the American Diabetes Association: Call 1-800-806-7801; Web site: www.diabetes.org/membership.

For more information about diabetes or ADA programs and services: Call 1-800-342-2383; E-mail: Customerservice@diabetes.org; Web site: www.diabetes.org.

To locate an ADA/NCQA recognized provider of quality diabetes care in your area: Call 1-703-549-1500, ext. 2202; Web site: www.diabetes.org/recognition/Physicians/ListAll.asp.

To find an ADA recognized education program in your area: Call 1-888-232-0822; Web site: www.diabetes.org/recognition/education.asp.

To find out about an important research project regarding type 2 diabetes: Web site: www.diabetes.org/ada/research.asp.

The American Dietetic Association
216 West Jackson Boulevard
Chicago, IL 60606
(312) 899-0040
www.eatright.org
The professional organization for registered dietitians. Also provides a wealth of information to the general public on nutrition to promote optimal health and well-being.

Division of Diabetes Translation, Centers for Disease Control and Prevention (CDC)
National Center for Chronic Disease Prevention and Health Promotion
TISB Mail Stop K-13
4770 Buford Highway, NE
Atlanta, GA 30341-3724
(404) 488-5080
Diabetes home page: www.cdc.gov/diabetes/ddthome.htm

An agency of the Public Health Service, Department of Health and Human Services. Its mission is to reduce the burden of diabetes in the United States. It supports diabetes control programs in numerous states; carries out state and national programs to assess the prevalence of diabetes; supports community-based preventive programs; coordinates federal activities concerned with translating research findings into clinical practice; among other activities. This group also publishes information for patients and primary care physicians.

eDiets
www.ediets.com

For $35 a month, this site offers advice for special dietary concerns, including nutrition for diabetes. You fill out a comprehensive questionnaire from which eDiets generates a diet, exercise program, and weekly shopping list. You keep an on-line record of what you eat and complete a weekly evaluation.

Glycemic Index Information
www.mendosa.com/gi.htm

This site provides the glycemic index of various foods to help manage blood glucose levels.

Indian Health Service (IHS)
IHS Headquarters West
Central Diabetes Program
5300 Homestead Road, NE
Albuquerque, NM 87110
(505) 837-4182
www.ihs.gov

An agency of the Public Health Service, this organization supports numerous programs serving Native Americans and Alaskans. These programs involve culturally accepted prevention and treatment methods for diabetes and its complications. IHS publishes culturally relevant publications, including nutrition guides, complication-specific educational materials, and guides for health care professionals.

International Diabetes Center (IDC)
5000 West 39th Street
Minneapolis, MN 55416
(612) 927-3393

IDC offers educational classes for people with diabetes and training programs for health professionals. It also publishes *Living Well with Diabetes*, a quarterly magazine for people with diabetes. Other publications include management and nutrition guides and guides for health care professionals.

International Diabetes Federation (IDF)
Rue DeFacqz B-1000
Brussels, Belgium
011-322-538-55-11
www.idf.org

IDF collaborates with more than 138 member associations in over 111 countries, the World Health Organization, and other affiliated organizations and individuals to ensure that people with diabetes receive quality care and education.

International Diabetic Athletes Association (IDAA)
1647 West Bethany Home Road #B
Phoenix, AZ 85015
(800)-898-IDAA
Fax: (602) 433-9331
www.diabetes-exercise.org

A nonprofit service organization whose members include people who participate in fitness activities at all levels and anyone interested in the relationship between diabetes and sports. The organization offers workshops, conferences, and events and has a regional network of chapters and support groups. The IDAA's quarterly newsletter, *The Challenge*, includes helpful articles about managing diabetes during athletic activities and articles about people with diabetes who compete in sports.

Joslin Diabetes Center
One Joslin Place
Boston, MA 02215
(617) 732-2415
www.joslin.harvard.edu

An international leader in diabetes research, treatment, and patient and professional education. It is affiliated with Harvard Medical School.

Juvenile Diabetes Foundation (JDF) International
432 Park Avenue South
New York, NY 10016-8013
(212) 889-7575 or (800) 223-1138
www.jdrf.org

A private, nonprofit organization with chapters throughout the world. The JDF raises funds to support research on the cause, cure, treatment, and prevention of diabetes and its complications. The organization sponsors numerous programs for health care professionals and scientists. It publishes a quarterly journal called *Countdown* and a series of patient education brochures about type 1 and type 2 diabetes.

National Diabetes Information Clearinghouse (NDIC)
1 Information Way
Bethesda, MD 20892-3560
www.chid.nih.gov

A service of the National Institute of Diabetes and Digestive and Kidney Diseases, which is the government's primary agency for diabetes research. The clearinghouse is an information, educational, and referral source for health professionals, people with diabetes, and the general public. NDIC publishes a variety of information on diabetes.

National Eye Institute (NEI)
2020 Vision Place
Bethesda, MD 20892
(301) 496-5248
www.nei.nih.gov

NEI is one of the National Institutes of Health. It supports research to develop treatments for diabetic eye disease. NEI's National Eye Health Education Program promotes public and professional awareness of the importance of early diagnosis and treatment of diabetic eye disease. NEI also publishes patient and professional education materials on diabetic eye disease, including patient literature, guides for health professionals, and education kits for community health workers and pharmacists.

National Institute of Diabetes and Digestive and Kidney Diseases (NIDDK)
1 Information Way
Bethesda, MD 20892
www.niddk.nih.gov

Conducts and supports research on kidney, urologic, blood, digestive, metabolic, and endocrine diseases, as well as on diabetes and nutrition. The NIDDK also provides a wealth of easy-to-read health information for the public.

National Kidney Foundation
30 East 33rd Street
New York, NY 10016
(800) 622-9010
www.kidney.org
Dedicated to improving the care and treatment of those afflicted with kidney and urinary tract disease through advances in detection, diagnosis, and treatment. Information for patients is available from the foundation.

WEB SITES

In addition to the Web sites mentioned above, here are other sites that may be helpful if you have diabetes, some of which may require an enrollment fee for use.

www.diabetes.com
Not to be confused with diabetes.org (the Web site of the American Diabetes Association), this site offers interactive tools, an expert columnist, answers from staff pharmacies, and a range of diabetic products and medications. Also available are articles covering a wide range of diabetes topics, including prevention, conventional and alternative treatments, tight blood glucose, and diet and fitness. Diabetes.com is a satellite health channel of PlanetRx.com, a health-information resource and on-line pharmacy.

www.diabeteslife.net
Sponsored by Roche Diagnostics, this site provides information on advances in diabetes treatment, information for parents about children with diabetes, patient education, living with diabetes, and community resources.

www.diabetesmanager.com
This Internet-based medical service provides individualized information to better control your diabetes based on your physician's prescription. It also assists physicians and other care providers in delivering intensive management to people with diabetes.

www.diabetesstation.org
A source for current information about living with diabetes, diabetes treatments, insulin pumps, insurance guidance, and more. There is also a message board on which you can post questions and messages.

www.diabeteswell.com
This site delivers a program that combines leading accepted practices for controlling glucose and preventing complications with dietary and fitness plans. You get on-line access to a team of physicians and experts who work with you and your doctor. In addition, you can try the program at no charge for ninety days with no obligation.

www.goodbloodsugar.com
A service of Islet Sheet Medical that provides resources to help you manage your diabetes. It gives information on the latest progress toward a cure, diabetes products, advice from experts, and links to other Web sites.

www.insulin-pumpers.org
Provides information and support for adults and children with diabetes and their families who are interested in insulin pump therapy.

www.niddk.nih.gov/health/diabetes/pubs/dmover/dmover.htm
Provided by the National Institute of Diabetes and Digestive and Kidney Disease, this site offers information on diabetes, its management, and future research efforts.

www.webmd.com
This leading medical site has a program called the Diabetes Resource Center, with which you can learn how to manage the disease and prevent its complications. Registering at WebMD makes you eligible to receive the site's free *Diabetes Newsletter*. Registration also gives you access to diabetes message boards, chat rooms, and other special events.

BOOKS

There are hundreds of books available on diabetes. Here are several recommended books that can help you learn more about the disease, as well as obtain guidance on nutrition, fitness, and treatments.

American Diabetes Association Complete Guide to Diabetes (New York:

Bantam Books, 1999). A comprehensive reference that provides information on the best self-care techniques and latest medical breakthroughs.

American Diabetes Association Diabetes Cookbook (Alexandria, VA: American Diabetes Association, 2000). This comprehensive and practical cookbook helps people with diabetes take control of their condition and live life to the fullest. Includes more than 100 beautifully illustrated recipes. Each recipe has a full nutritional analysis.

The Diabetes Carbohydrate & Calorie Counter by Annette B. Natow et al. (New York: Pocket Books, 1991). This reference includes 3,000 alphabetical entries of convenience and home-cooked foods (with calorie, carbohydrate, sugar, and fat counts), diet plans, and more.

The Diabetes Carbohydrate and Fat Gram Guide by Lea Ann Holzmeister (Alexandria, VA: American Diabetes Association, 2000). A guide to the carbohydrate and fat content of the foods you eat, whether you're cooking at home, eating out, or using packaged foods.

Diabetes for Dummies by Alan L. Rubin, M.D. (Foster City, CA: IDG Books Worldwide, 1999). Covers diabetes prevention and treatment, motivation, fitness, drug treatments, and advice for healthy living. Dr. Rubin has also written *Diabetes Cookbook for Dummies* (Foster City, CA: Hungry Minds, 2000), which includes 112 tasty recipes that take a half hour or less of preparation, plus cooking time.

Diabetes Meal Planning Made Easy: How to Put the Food Pyramid to Work for Your Busy Lifestyle by Hope S. Warshaw (Alexandria, VA: American Diabetes Association, 2000). An essential guide to menu planning that uses the easy-to-understand food guide pyramid. Also included is helpful information about nutrition for people with diabetes.

The Diabetic Athlete by Sheri Colberg, Ph.D. (Champaign, IL: Human Kinetics, 2000). The only book on the market that gives athletes and dedicated fitness enthusiasts with type 1 and type 2 diabetes the practical information they need to better manage their diabetes. The book covers the basics of exercise, metabolism, nutrition, and supplements. Dr. Colberg is a diabetic athlete.

Guide to Carbohydrate Counting: A Simple Meal-Planning Method for People with Diabetes (Minneapolis, MN Fairview, 2001). With this book, you can learn more about carbohydrate counting, one of the most popular meal-planning tools available for people with diabetes.

Natural Treatments for Diabetes by Kathleen Head, N.D. (Roseville, CA: Prima, 2000). Provides science-backed information on a variety of nutritional and herbal treatments for diabetes.

The Official Pocket Guide to Diabetic Exchanges (Alexandria, VA: American

Diabetic Association, 1998). This handy reference is a pocket-sized quick guide to the American Diabetes Association and American Dietetic Association's exchange lists for meal planning.

DIABETES SELF-CARE SUPPLIES

The best source of information about types of insulin, insulin delivery products, aids for injection and self-monitoring, and other diabetes care products is *Buyer's Guide to Diabetes Supplies*, published each year in *Diabetes Forecast*. To order a copy, call your local American Diabetes Association chapter, or the American Diabetes Association at (800) 232-3472.

References

STOPPING A SILENT KILLER

American Academy of Family Physicians. 1998. Do I have diabetes? *American Family Physician*, October 15. On-line: www.findarticles.com.

American Diabetes Association. 1999. *American Diabetes Association Complete Guide to Diabetes.* New York: Bantam Books.

———. 2001. Diabetes info. www.diabetes.org.

Broida, M. 2001. Cow's milk and type 1 diabetes. www.tnp.com.

Diabetes. 2001. www.webmd.com.

Diabetes overview. 2001. www.medscape.com.

Diabetes statistics. 2001. www.webmd.com.

Morgan, P. 1998. The silent epidemic. *Prevention*, March, pp. 86–93, 168.

Schardt, D., et al. 2000. What is diabetes? www.diabetes.com.

What is type 2 diabetes? 2001. www.diabetesmanager.com.

UNMASKING TROUBLE:
HOW YOUR DOCTOR DIAGNOSES DIABETES

Diagnosis: diabetes. 2001. www.webmd.com.

For people with diabetes. 2001. www.webmd.com.

Fukunishi, I., et al. 1998. Perception and utilization of social support in diabetic control. *Diabetes Research and Clinical Practice* 41: 207–11.

Kluger, J. 2000. The diabetes explosion. *Time*, September 4, p. 58.

Landis, B. J. 1996. Uncertainty, spiritual well-being, and psychosocial adjustment. *Issues in Mental Health Nursing* 17: 217–31.

What are the diagnostic tests for type 2 diabetes? 2001. www.webmd.com.

Zaret, B. L. 1997. *The Yale University School of Medicine Patient's Guide to Medical Tests*. Boston: Houghton Mifflin.

YOU MAY HAVE DIABETES, BUT YOU DON'T HAVE TO GET ITS LIFE-THREATENING COMPLICATIONS

American Diabetes Association. 1999. *American Diabetes Association Complete Guide to Diabetes*. New York: Bantam Books.
———. 2001. Diabetes info. www.diabetes.org.

CHOOSING QUALITY CAREGIVERS

American Diabetes Association. 1999. *American Diabetes Association Complete Guide to Diabetes*. New York: Bantam Books.
———. 2000. Proof: American Diabetes Association program improves patient care. June 10. News release.
Lally, E. 1992. Doctor shopping '92. *Prevention*, April, pp. 42–49, 120.
Shealey, T. 1986. How to find a great doctor. *Prevention*, April, pp. 123–31.

MEDICAL TESTS AND MEDICATIONS THAT CAN SAVE YOUR LIFE

All about insulin. 1994. *Diabetes Forecast* 47: 57–59.
American Diabetes Association. 2001. Buyer's guide—insulin. www.diabetes.org.
———. 2001. Update regarding discontinuation of animal-source insulins. www.diabetes.org.
D'Arrigo, T. 1999. Cholesterol: the good, the bad, and the ugly. *Diabetes Forecast*, October 1, pp. 54–58.
Guthrie, D. W., et al. 1999. *The Diabetes Sourcebook: Today's Methods and Ways to Give Yourself the Best Care*. Lincolnwood, IL: Lowell House.
High blood pressure. 2001. www.webmd.com.
Hirsch, I. B. 1998. Why good people get poor diabetes care. www.diabetes.org.
Standards of care. 2001. www.webmd.com.
Stenger, A. 1993. New guidelines for hypertension. *The Physician and Sportsmedicine* 21: 55–56.
Warren-Boulton, E. 1999. An update on the primary care management of type 2 diabetes. *The Nurse Practitioner* 24: 14, 16, 19.

EAT TO BEAT DIABETES: UNDERSTANDING THE ROLE OF NUTRITION

American Diabetes Association. 2001. Eating healthy basics. www.diabetes.org.

———. 2001. Nutrition recommendations and principles for people with diabetes mellitus. Position statement.

Henkel, J. 1999. Sugar substitutes: Americans opt for sweetness and light. *FDA Consumer.* November–December. www.fda.gov.

Kleiner, S. M., and M. Greenwood-Robinson. 1998. *High Performance Nutrition.* New York: John Wiley.

Nutrition recommendations and principles for people with diabetes. 1994. *Diabetes Care* 17: 519–22.

Nutrition recommendations for nutritional management of patients with diabetes mellitus. 2000. *European Journal of Clinical Nutrition* 54: 353–55.

Nuttall, F. Q., et al. Nutrition and the management of type 2 diabetes. *The Journal of Family Practice* 47: S45–53.

Sizer, F., and E. Whitney. 1997. *Nutrition Concepts and Controversies.* 7th ed. Belmont, CA: West/Wadsworth.

THE EXERCISE CONNECTION

American Diabetes Association. 2000. Diabetes mellitus and exercise. Position statement.

Eriksson, J. 1999. Exercise and the treatment of type 2 diabetes mellitus: an update. *Sports Medicine* 27: 381–91.

Eriksson, J., et al. 1997. Resistance training in the treatment of non-insulin-dependent diabetes. *International Journal of Sports Medicine* 18: 242–46.

Honkola, A., et al. 1997. Resistance training improves the metabolic profile in individuals with type 2 diabetes. *Acta Diabetologica* 34: 245–48.

Soukup, J. T., et al. 1993. A review of the effects of resistance training for individuals with diabetes mellitus. *The Diabetes Educator* 19: 307–12.

White, R., et al. 1999. Exercise in diabetes management. *The Physician and Sportsmedicine.* April. www.physsportmed.com.

STEP ONE: FOLLOW A HEALING, HEALTHY DIET

Aitken, G. 1997. Nutrition and diabetes: putting guidelines into practice. *British Journal of Nursing* 6: 1035–38.

American Diabetes Association. 2001. Eating healthy with the diabetes food guide pyramid as your guide. www.diabetes.org.

———. 2001. Glycemic index. www.diabetes.org.

Arcement, P. S. 1999. Carbohydrate counting in diabetes meal planning. *Home Healthcare Nurse* 17: 425–28.

Barrier, P. 1994. Goodbye to the diabetic diet. *Nation's Business*, November 1, p. 86.

Benedict, M. 1999. Carbohydrate counting: tips for simplifying diabetes education. *Health Care Food & Nutrition Focus* 16: 6–9.

Carbo counting. 1995. *Diabetes Forecast* 48: 30–37.

Chan, P., et al. 2000. A double-blind placebo-controlled study of the effectiveness and tolerability of oral stevioside in human hypertension. *British Journal of Clinical Pharmacology* 50: 215–20.

Counting carbohydrates. 2001. www.diabeteswell.com.

Daly, A., et al. 1995. Carbohydrate counting: getting started. Chicago: American Dietetics Association.

Daly, A., et al. 1997. Tales from carbo land. *Diabetes Forecast* 50: 34–39.

D'Arrigo, T. 1999. Cholesterol: the good, the bad, and the ugly. *Diabetes Forecast* 52: 54–58.

Delaney, L. 1992. Reverse Diabetes. *Prevention*, July, pp. 33–41, 98–104.

Diet. The glycemic index. 1999. *Harvard Health Letter* 24: 7.

50 top nutrition tips. 1996. *Nursing* 26: 55–56.

Foster-Powell, K., et al. 1995. International tables of glycemic index. *American Journal of Clinical Nutrition* 62: 871S–90S.

Frost, G. 2000. The relevance of the glycemic index to our understanding of dietary carbohydrate. *Diabetic Medicine* 17: 336–45.

Garg, A. 1994. High-monounsaturated fat diet for diabetic patients: is it time to change the current dietary recommendations? *Diabetes Care* 17: 242–46.

Gillespie, S. J. 1998. Using carbohydrate counting in clinical diabetes practice. *Journal of the American Dietetic Association* 98: 897–905.

Gumbiner, B. 1999. The treatment of obesity in type 2 diabetes mellitus. *Primary Care* 26: 869–83.

Henry, S. 1995. Banish blood-sugar blues. *Prevention*, February, pp. 85–90.

Holler, H. J. 1991. Understanding the use of the exchange lists for meal planning. *The Diabetes Educator* 17: 474–84.

———. 1995. Your updated exchange lists: greater choices, more flexibility. *Diabetes Forecast* 48: 75–77.

Jeppesen, P. B., et al. 2000. Stevioside acts directly on pancreatic beta cells to secrete insulin: actions independent of cyclic adenosine monophosphate and adenoside triphosphate-sensitive K+-channel activity. *Metabolism* 49: 208–14.

Mann, D. 2000. Successful dieting diabetics do well. *WebMD Medical News.* www.webmd.com.

Miller, J. C. 1994. Importance of glycemic index in diabetes. *American Journal of Clinical Nutrition* 59: 747S–52S.

Morris, K. L., et al. 1999. Glycemic index, cardiovascular disease, and obesity. *Nutrition Review* 57: 273–76.

Nidus Information Services, Inc. 1998. Diabetes diet. www.webmd.com.

Spollet, G. 1997. Diet strategies in the treatment of non-insulin-dependent diabetes mellitus. *Lippincott's Primary Care Practice* 1: 295–304.

U.S. Department of Agriculture. 1992. *Home and Garden Bulletin* 252.

Webb, R. 1997. Quick cooking. *Diabetes Forecast* 50: 32–36.

Wolever, T. M. 1997. The glycemic index: flogging a dead horse? *Diabetes Care* 20: 452–56.

STEP TWO: DRIVE DIABETES INTO RETREAT WITH NATURAL REMEDIES

American Diabetes Association. 1996. Magnesium supplementation in the treatment of diabetes. Consensus statement.

American Society of Bariatric Physicians. 2000. What is obesity? www.asbp.org/obesity.htm.

Anderson, J. W., et al. 1999. Effects of psyllium on glucose and serum lipid responses in men with type 2 diabetes and hypercholesterolemia. *American Journal of Clinical Nutrition* 70: 466–73.

Badmaev, V., et al. 1999. Vanadium: a review of its potential role in the fight against diabetes. *Journal of Alternative and Complementary Medicine* 5: 273–91.

Bailey, C. J., et al. 1989. Traditional plant medicines as treatments for diabetes. *Diabetes Care* 12: 553–64.

Barilla, J. 1999. Get a grip on glucose. *Better Nutrition*, December. www.findarticles.com.

Basu, S., et al. 2000. Conjugated linoleic acid induces lipid peroxidation in humans. *FEBS Letter* 468: 33–36.

Bauman, W. A., et al. 2000. Increased intake of calcium reverses vitamin B_{12} malabsorption induced by metformin. *Diabetes Care* 23: 1227–31.

Berman, B. M., et al. 1999. Complementary and alternative medicine: herbal therapies for diabetes. *Journal of the Association for Academic Minority Physicians* 10: 10–14.

Blostein-Fujii, A., et al. 1997. Short-term zinc supplementation in women with non-insulin-dependent diabetes mellitus. *American Journal of Clinical Nutrition* 66: 639–42.

Bran buds gets FDA endorsement. 1998. *Evansville Courier*, February 18, p. C–9.

Broadhurst, C. L., et al. 2000. Insulin-like biological activity of culinary and medicinal plant aqueous extracts in vivo. *Journal of Agriculture and Food Chemistry* 48: 849–52.

Bursell, S. E., et al. 1999. High-dose vitamin E supplementation normalizes retinal blood flow and creatinine clearance in patients with type 1 diabetes. *Diabetes Care* 22: 1245–51.

Cam, M. C., et al. 2000. Mechanisms of vanadium action: insulin-mimetic or insulin-enhancing agent? *Canadian Journal of Physiology and Pharmacology* 78: 829–47.

Can vitamin E help stop retinopathy? 1998. *Medical Post* 34: 24.

Ceriello, A., et al. Vitamin E reduction of protein glycosylation in diabetes. *Diabetes Care* 14: 68–72.

Cesa, F. 1990. The use of vegetable fibers in the treatment of pregnancy diabetes and/or excessive weight gain during pregnancy. *Minerva Ginecologica* 42: 271–74.

Chromium—little known, seldom used, but very essential to health. 1993. *Nutrition Health Review*, Spring, 10.

Conjugated linoleic acid overview. Professional monographs: herbal, mineral, vitamin, nutraceuticals. 2001. *Intramedicine*, March 1.

Cunningham, J. J. 1998. Micronutrients as nutriceutical intervention in diabetes mellitus. *Journal of the American College of Nutrition* 17: 7–10.

D'Arrigo, T. 2000. Reeling in answers about fish oil. www.diabetes.org.

De Valk, H. W. 1999. Magnesium in diabetes mellitus. *The Netherlands Journal of Medicine* 54: 139–46.

Duke, J. A. 1997. *The Green Pharmacy*. Emmaus, PA: Rodale Press.

Eder, R. 1999. Alpha-lipoic acid and diabetics. *Drug Store News*, September 27. www.findarticles.com.

Faure, P., et al. 1995. Lipid peroxidation in insulin-dependent diabetic patients with early retina degenerative lesions: effects of an oral zinc supplementation. *European Journal of Clinical Nutrition* 49: 282–88.

Fox, G. N., et al. 1998. Chromium picolinate supplementation for diabetes mellitus. *The Journal of Family Practice* 46: 83–86.

Fremerman, S. 1998. Alpha-lipoic acid. *Natural Health*, September/October. www.findarticles.com.

Fujioka, T., et al. 1983. Clinical study of cardiac arrhythmias using a 24-hour continuous electrocardiographic recorder (5th report)—antiarrhythmic action of coenzyme Q10 in diabetics. *The Tohoku Journal of Experimental Medicine* 141: 453–63.

Geraci, R. 1999. Malegrams: supplements: alpha-lipoic acid. *Men's Health*, July, p. 34.

Harder, P. 1998. Alpha-lipoic acid: energy at the cellular level. *Better Nutrition*, April. www.findarticles.com.

Houseknecht, K. L., et al. 1998. Dietary conjugated linoleic acid normalizes impaired glucose tolerance in the Zucker diabetic fatty fa/fa rat. *Biochemical and Biophysical Research Communications* 244: 678–82.

Jain, S. K., et al. 1996. The effect of modest vitamin E supplementation on lipid peroxidation products and other cardiovascular risk factors in diabetic patients. *Lipids* 31: S87–90.

Jain, S. K., et al. 1996. Effect of modest vitamin E supplementation on blood glycated hemoglobin and triglyceride levels and red cell indices in type 1 diabetic patients. *Journal of the American College of Clinical Nutrition* 15: 458–61.

Kahuda, T., et al. 1996. Hypoglycemic effect of extracts from Lagerstroemia speciosa L. leaves in genetically diabetic KK-AY mice. *Bioscience, Biotechnology, and Biochemistry* 60: 204–08.

Kelly, G. S. 2000. Insulin resistance: lifestyle and nutritional interventions. *Alternative Medicine Review* 5: 109–32.

Kunisaki, M., et al. 1990. Effects of vitamin E administration on platelet function in diabetes mellitus. *Diabetes Research* 14: 37–42.

Lavalle, J. B. 1999. Using dietary supplements to maintain ocular health in diabetic patients. *Drug Store News*, March 15. www.findarticles.com.

Linday, L. A. 1997. Trivalent chromium and the diabetes prevention program. *Medical Hypotheses* 49: 47–49.

Madar, Z., et al. 1988. Glucose-lowering effect of fenugreek in non-insulin dependent diabetics. *European Journal of Clinical Nutrition* 42: 51–54.

McBride, J. 2000. Cinnamon extracts boost insulin sensitivity. *Agricultural Research*, July. www.ars.usda.gov.

McCarty, M. F. 1999. Can correction of sub-optimal coenzyme Q10 status improve beta cell function in type II diabetics? *Medical Hypotheses* 52: 397–400.

Miyake, Y., et al. 1999. Effect of treatment with 3-hydroxy-3-methylglutaryl coenzyme A reductase inhibitors on serum coenzyme Q10 in diabetic patients. *Arzneimittelforschung* 49: 324–29.

Montori, V. M. 2000. Fish oil supplementation in type 2 diabetes: a quantitative systemic review. *Diabetes Care* 23: 1407–15.

More vitamin E? 1997. *Industry Week*, March 3, p. 24.

Morelli, J. 2000. Some diabetics buck tradition and turn to herbs. *WebMD Medical News*. www.webmd.com.

Morelli, V., et al. 2000. Alternative treatments: part I. Depression, diabetes, obesity. *American Family Physician* 62: 1051–60.

Morgan, P. 1998. The silent epidemic. *Prevention*, March, pp. 86–93, 168.

Mozersky, R. P. 1999. Herbal products and supplemental nutrients used in the management of diabetes. *Journal of the American Osteopathic Association* 99: S4–9.

Munson, M. 1995. Sink diabetes. *Prevention*, May, pp. 26–27.

Murakami, C., et al. 1993. Screening of plant constituents for effect on glucose transport activity in Ehrlich ascites tumour cells. *Chemical and Pharmaceutical Bulletin* 41: 2129–31.

Murray, M. T. 1996. *Encyclopedia of Nutritional Substances*. Rocklin, CA: Prima.

Nicolosi, R. J., et al. 1997. Dietary conjugated linoleic acid reduces plasma lipoproteins and early aortic atherosclerosis in hypercholesterolemic hamsters. *Artery* 22: 266–77.

O'Brien, S. F., et al. 1995. Absence of increased susceptibility of LDL to oxidation in type 1 diabetics. *Diabetes Research and Clinical Practice* 30: 195–203.

Paolisso, G., et al. 1993. Pharmacologic doses of vitamin E improve insulin action in healthy subjects and non-insulin-dependent diabetic subjects. *American Journal of Clinical Nutrition* 57: 650–56.

Passwater, R. A. 1992. *Chromium Picolinate: Breakthrough in Sports Nutrition*. New Canaan, CT: Keats Publishing.

———. 1995. *Lipoic Acid: The Metabolic Antioxidant*. New Canaan, CT: Keats Publishing.

Persaud, S. J., et al. 1999. Gymnema sylvestre stimulates insulin release in vitro by increased membrane permeability. *Journal of Endocrinology* 163: 207–12.

Rodriguez-Moran, M., et al. 1998. Lipid- and glucose-lowering efficacy of plantago psyllium in type 1 diabetes. *Journal of Diabetes Complications* 12: 273–78.

Shanmugasundarum, E. R. 1990. Use of gymnema sylvestre leaf extract in the control of blood glucose in insulin-dependent diabetes mellitus. *Journal of Ethnopharmacology* 30: 281–94.

Sharma, R. D., et al. 1990. Effect of fenugreek seeds on blood glucose and serum lipids in type 1 diabetes. *European Journal of Clinical Nutrition* 44: 301–06.

Singh, R. B., et al. 1999. Effect of hydrosoluble coenzyme Q10 on blood pressures and insulin resistance in hypertensive patients with coronary artery disease. *Journal of Human Hypertension* 13: 203–08.

Sotaniemi, E. A., et al. 1995. Ginseng therapy in non-insulin-dependent diabetic patients. *Diabetes Care* 18: 1373–75.

Stene, L. C., et al. 2000. Use of cod liver oil during pregnancy associated with lower risk of type 1 diabetes in the offspring. *Diabetologica* 43: 1093–98.

Truitt, A., et al. 1999. Antiplatelet effects of conjugated linoleic acid isomers. *Biochimica et Biophysica Acta* 1438: 239–46.

Tsuboyama-Kasaoka, N. 2000. Conjugated linoleic acid supplementation reduces adipose tissue by apoptosis and develops lipodystrophy in mice. *Diabetes Care* 49: 1534–42.

Tutuncu, N. B., et al. 1998. Reversal of defective nerve conduction with vitamin E supplementation in type 2 diabetes: a preliminary study. *Diabetes Care* 21: 1915–18.

West, D. B., et al. 1998. Effects of conjugated linoleic acid on body fat and energy metabolism in the mouse. *American Journal of Physiology* 275: R667–72.

Will, J. C., et al. 1996. Does diabetes mellitus increase the requirement for vitamin C? *Nutrition Reviews* 54: 193–202.

Ziegler, J. 1989. A sweet spice for diabetics: cinnamon may boost the effects of insulin. *American Health*, November, 96–97.

STEP THREE: TEST YOUR BLOOD SUGAR REGULARLY

American Diabetes Association. 2000. Buyer's guide—products for treating reactions. www.diabetes.org.

———. 2000. Buyer's guide—blood glucose monitors and data management. www.diabetes.org.

———. 1999. Statement regarding the FDA Advisory Committee's recommendations on GlucoWatch. www.diabetes.org.

———. 1996. Tight diabetes control. www.diabetes.org.

Bloom, A. 1998. Tips for your fingertips: here are 5 suggestions for improving your fingerstick technique. *Diabetes Forecast* 51: 70–72.

Cygnus. 2001. GlucoWatch Biographer. www.cyng.com.

Diabetes self-testing: Simple tests you do yourself can help you care for your diabetes and feel better. 1996. *Diabetes Forecast* 49: 75–77.

Know your blood sugar numbers. 2001. www.webmd.com.

Reach your blood sugar goal. 2001. www.webmd.com.

STEP FOUR: GET FIT TO FIGHT DIABETES

Albright, A., et al. 2000. American College of Sports Medicine position stand: exercise and type 2 diabetes. *Medicine and Science and Sports and Exercise* 32: 1345–60.

American Diabetes Association. Frequently asked questions: exercise and diabetes. www.diabetes.org.

Borg, G. 1982. Psychophysical bases of perceived exertion. *Medicine and Science in Sports and Exercise* 14: 377–81.

Colberg, S. R. 2000. Use of clinical practice recommendations for exercise by individuals with type 1 diabetes. *The Diabetes Educator* 26: 265–71.

Durak, E. P., et al. 1990. Randomized crossover study of effect of resistance training. *Diabetes Care* 13: 1039–43.

Ivy, J. L., et al. 1999. Prevention and treatment of non-insulin-dependent diabetes mellitus. *Exercise and Sports Science Reviews* 27: 1–35.

Krucoff, C. 1995. Running on insulin. *Saturday Evening Post*, July 17, p. 14.

Mihalik, M. 1986. Get fit to fight diabetes. *Prevention*, July, pp. 93–98.

Scheiner, G. 1994. The best exercise (for diabetics). *Diabetes Forecast* 47: 46–50.

———. 1996. Pace yourself. *Diabetes Forecast* 49: 32–36.

———. 1994. When the workout is out. *Diabetes Forecast* 47: 42–45.

Soukup, J. T., et al. 1994. Resistance training guidelines for individuals with diabetes. *The Diabetes Educator* 20: 129–37.

Verity, L. S., et al. 1998. Getting fit with fits and starts. *Diabetes Forecast* 51: 74–78.

Walberg-Henriksson, H., et al. Exercise in the management of non-insulin-dependent diabetes mellitus. *Sports Medicine* 25: 25–35.

White, R., et al. 1999. Exercising with diabetes. *The Physician and Sportsmedicine*. April. www.physsportsmed.com.

Zinker, B. A. 1999. Nutrition and exercise in individuals with diabetes. *Clinics in Sports Medicine* 18: vii–viii, 585–606.

STEP FIVE: TAKE MEDICINE IF YOUR DOCTOR PRESCRIBES IT

American Diabetes Association. 1999. *American Diabetes Association Complete Guide to Diabetes*. New York: Bantam Books.

———. 2000. Buyer's guide—insulin delivery. www.diabetes.org.

———. 1996. Buyer's guide—syringes. www.diabetes.org.

———. 2000. Buyer's guide—urine testing. www.diabetes.org.

———. 2000. Continuous subcutaneous insulin infusion. Position statement.

———. 2001. Controlling diabetes with class. www.diabetes.org.

———. 2001. Diabetes info. www.diabetes.org.

———. 2001. Inhaled insulin study results promising. www.diabetes.org.

———. 2001. Oral diabetes medications. www.diabetes.org.

———. 2001. Q & A regarding Starlix. www.diabetes.org.

———. 1999. What you need to known about pioglitazone hydrochloride (Actos), a new type 2 diabetes oral medication. www.diabetes.org.
Ammerman, D. 1999. The life-saving power of aspirin. www.diabetes.org.
Bogosian, J. 1996. Insulin insights: separate the myth from the truth and you may not be so opposed to insulin therapy to control your type II diabetes. *Diabetes Forecast* 49: 54–57.
David, S. 1999. Advanced in therapy for type 2 diabetes. *Patient Care Archive*, October 15. www.pdr.net.
DeCherney, G. S. 1997. Time for a tune-up? *Diabetes Forecast* 50: 22–24.
Ehmann, K. 1995. Over 60 & newly diagnosed. *Diabetes Forecast* 48: 34–38.
Foster, R. 2001. Starlix offers a new approach to type 2 diabetes. www.pharminfo.com.
Frazzita-Luerssen, M., et al. 1997. Basal rates. *Diabetes Forecast* 50: 45.
Hirsch, I. B. 1999. Type 1 diabetes mellitus and the use of flexible insulin. *American Family Physician*, November 15. www.findarticles.com.
Insulin use and type 2 diabetes. 1999. *Medical Post* 35: pp. Q1–Q8.
Jeffrey, S. 1999. American Diabetes Association: an ASA a day can keep doctors away for diabetics. *Medical Post*, July 7. www.elibrary.com.
Medical Economics Company. 2001. *The PDR Family Guide to Prescription Drugs*. www.pdr.net.
Oral medications. 2001. www.glucovance.com.
Patten, B. C., et al. 1999. Out on a limb? should type 2s use insulin pumps? www.diabetes.com.
Riddle, M. C., et al. 1999. Are you overdue for insulin? www.diabetes.org.
Robertson, C. 2000. Understanding your insulin prescription. June. www.goodbloodsugar.com.
Schwartz, S. L. 1998. Double your injections; tighten your control. *Diabetes Forecast* 51: 52–54.
Sherwin, R. 1996. Pill time. www.diabetes.org.

STEP SIX: DEFEAT STRESS WITH POSITIVE LIVING

Basco, M. R. 1998. Perfectionism and diabetes care. *Diabetes Spectrum* 11: 43–48.
Berlin, I., et al. 1997. Phobic symptoms, particularly the fear of blood and injury, are associated with poor glycemic control in type 1 diabetic adults. *Diabetes Care* 20: 176.
Bolderman, K. M. 1996. Faithful fasting (with diabetes). *Diabetes Forecast* 49: 48–50.
D'Arrigo, T. 1999. Cognitive therapy can help type 2s. www.diabetes.org.
———. 2000. Stress and diabetes. www.diabetes.org.

Edelstein, J., et al. 1985. The influence of the family on the control of diabetes. *Social Science & Medicine* 21: 541–44.

Gilden, J. L., et al. 1992. Diabetes support groups improve health care of older diabetic patients. *Journal of the American Geriatrics Society* 40: 147–50.

Glasgow, R. E., et al. 1999. In diabetes care, moving from compliance to adherence is not enough. *Diabetes Care*, December. www.findarticles.com.

Green, L., et al. 2000. Fears and phobias in people with diabetes. *Diabetes/Metabolism Research and Reviews* 16: 287–93.

Griffith, L. S., et al. 1990. Life stress and social support in diabetes: association with glycemic control. *International Journal of Psychiatry in Medicine* 20: 365–72.

Hall, L. L. 1997. The things that go bump in the mind. *FDA Consumer*, March 1. www.elibrary.com.

Kawakami, N., et al. 2000. Job strain, social support in the workplace, and haemoglobin A1c in Japanese men. *Occupational and Environmental Medicine* 57: 805–09.

La Greca, A. M., et al. 1995. I get by with a little help from family and friends: adolescents' support for diabetes care. *Journal of Pediatric Psychology* 20: 449–76.

Leo, J. 1986. Talk is as good as a pill. *Time*, May 26, p. 60.

Lustman, P. J. 2000. Depression and poor glycemic control. *Diabetes Care*, July. www.findarticles.com.

Lustman, P. J., et al. 1997. Identifying depression in adults with diabetes. www.diabetes.org.

Lustman, P. J., et al. 1998. Depression: beyond the blues. www.diabetes.org.

Maxwell, A. E., et al. 1992. Effects of a social support group, as an adjunct to diabetes training, on metabolic control and psychosocial outcomes. *The Diabetes Educator* 18: 303–09.

Mengel, M. B., et al. 1990. The relationship of family dynamics/social support to patient functioning in IDDM patients on intensive insulin therapy. *Diabetes Research and Clinical Practice* 9: 149–62.

Michaud, E. 1998. Do you have the miracle healer in you? *Prevention*, December, pp. 106–113, 163.

Neal, A. 1998. The benefits of religious practice. *Saturday Evening Post*, March 1, p. 38.

Online support: chronically ill patients report benefits, high levels of satisfaction. 2000. *Disease Management Advisor* 6: 149, 158–61.

Rapaport, W. S. 1999. Diabetes in the family. www.diabetes.org.

Ruggiero, L., et al. 1990. Impact of social support and stress on compliance in women with gestational diabetes. *Diabetes Care* 13: 441–43.

Samuel-Hodge, C. D., et al. 2000. Influences on day-to-day self-management of type 2 diabetes among African-American women: spirituality, the multi-caregiver role, and other social context factors. *Diabetes Care* 23: 928–33.

Schafer, L. C., et al. 1986. Supportive and nonsupportive family behaviors: relationships to adherence and metabolic control in persons with type 1 diabetes. *Diabetes Care* 9: 179–85.

Sharpe, J. 1999. Psychological adjustment when diabetes is diagnosed. *Community Nurse* 5: 17–18.

Shenkel, R. J., et al. 1985–1986. Importance of "significant others" in predicting cooperation with diabetic regimen. *International Journal of Psychiatry in Medicine* 15: 149–55.

Stocker, S. 1995. 7 signs of a good therapist. *Prevention*, August, pp. 80–85.

Stress: what stress does to diabetes control. 1995. *Diabetes Forecast* 48: 56–58.

Talbot, F. 2000. A review of the relationship between depression and diabetes in adults: Is there a link? *Diabetes Care*, October. www.findarticles.com.

Toth, E. L. 1992. Description of a diabetes support group: lessons for diabetes caregivers. *Diabetic Medicine* 9: 773–78.

Index

abdominal fat, 14, 15, 135
acesulfame K, 67
acetyl-l-carniline, 150 (table)
Actos, 199–200
advanced glycated end products (AGEs), 49, 115–16, 121
aerobic dancing, 53, 73
aerobic exercise, 73–76, 109
  benefits of, 74–76
  setting up a program of, 169–74
African Americans, 12, 13, 19
age, and diabetes risk, 7, 16
Aitken, Gillian, 71
albumin, 115
alcoholic beverages, 69–71, 105, 107
S-allylcysteine sulfoxide, 143
alpha-glucosidase inhibitors, 197–98
alpha-lipoic acid, 119–21, 149 (table), 151
alphacarotene, 114
alternative care practitioner, 42–43
Amaryl, 194, 196 (table)
American Association of Diabetes Educators, 41
American Diabetes Association (ADA), 20–21, 39, 95
American Indians, 12, 13, 19
American Society of Bariatric Physicians, 106
amino acids, 63, 131–34, 147, 150 (table)
amputation, 29, 37 (table)
anemia, 124
angina, 29
animal-source insulins, 56
antibodies, 8
antidepressants, 213–14
antifungal cream, 37 (table)
antioxidants, 9, 16, 113, 119–23, 149 (table)
antiplatelet drug, 203–4
anxiety, 76, 212
appetite, 100, 212
  loss of, 161
aquatic exercise, 170
L-arginine, 132, 150 (table)
arm exercises, 54
arms, discomfort in, 165
arteries, 30, 77

arthernoma, 30
Asian Americans, 12, 13, 19
L-asparaginase, 9
aspartame, 67
aspirin therapy, 203–4
at-home self-monitoring kits, 153
atherosclerosis, 28–29, 77
Ativan, 216
autoimmune response, 6, 8
automatic injector, 190
autonomic neuropathy, 54
Avandia, 199–200

B cells, 6
B complex vitamins, 123–25, 149 (table)
baked goods, 62, 64, 65
banaba plant, 141
basal dose, 189–90
Beck, Aaron, 214
Bender, Lori, 109–11
benzodiazepines, 216
beta-carotene, 114
beta cells, 4–5, 6, 7, 8, 9, 67, 122, 209
bicycling, 54, 73
biguanides, 195–97
bilberry, 139, 150 (table), 151
bioflavonoids, 151
biotin, 123
bladder control, 33, 34
bladder infection, 4 (table)
blood clotting, 75
blood fats, 12, 77
blood pressure, 68–69, 123
   high. *See* high blood pressure
   normal and high, ranges of, 31 (table)
   See also high blood pressure
blood pressure exam, scheduling, 51 (table)
blood sugar (glucose), 63

   exercise causing problems with, 166–69
   ideal ranges of, for diabetics, 154–55
   levels of, 94
   reducing level of, by diet and exercise, 74, 76, 100–103, 121
   self-monitoring of, 153–62
   stress and, 208–9
   vitamin E and, 117–18
blood sugar (glucose) tests, 10, 17, 46
   for diagnosing diabetes, 24–27
   feelings of depression after, 158
   scheduling, 51 (table)
blood vessels, 5
   disease of, 119
bolus dose, 189–90
bones, 78, 126
Borg scale, 172–73
bovine serum albumin (BSA), 8
bowel control, 33
brain, 29
breast-feeding, 60
breath
   odor, fruity, 161
   shortness of, 165
breathing exercises, 210
breathing problems, 161

caffeine, 69
calcium, 108, 126–27, 149 (table)
calisthenics, 73
calories
   daily requirement, calculating, 82–83
   distributing among food sources, 83–86
   reducing, to lose weight, 105
candy, 62
capillaries, 75
carbohydrates, 61–62, 99
   conversion to glucose, 94
   counting, 94–95, 98 (table)

daily need for, calculating, 83–84
refined, 15
simple and complex, 62
cardiac complications, 122–23
cardiomyopathy, 123
cardiovascular status, and choice of exercise, 52–53
caregivers, choosing, 38–43
L-carniline, 150 (table)
L-carnitine, 133
carotenoids, 114
cataracts, 32
cells
  injury to, from free radicals, 8–9
  membranes of, 11
  response to insulin, 5
Centers for Disease Control and Prevention, 22
cereals, 62
certified diabetes educator (CDE), 22, 41
chair exercises, 54
chemical exposure, and diabetes, 9
chest, discomfort or pain in, 29, 165
children, diabetes in, 16, 180
chlorpropamide, 194
cholesterol, 28, 64
  dietary, 107
  HDL, 47 (table), 64, 106–7
  LDL, 47 (table), 64, 75, 77, 107, 116
  reducing, with diet, 106–7
  risk levels, 46, 47 (table)
  types of, 64
chromium, 127–28, 139, 149 (table)
cinnamon, 140
circulation, 75
  in extremities, 29, 52
  impaired, 34, 54, 183 (table)
circulatory status, and choice of exercise, 52–53, 183 (table)
cod liver oil, 138

coenzyme Q10 (CoQ10), 121–23, 149 (table)
cognitive behavior therapy (CBT), 214
Colberg, Sheri, 182
cold feet, 52
combination therapy, 202–3
complications of diabetes, 28–37
  prevention and treatment of, 36–37 (table)
concentration, poor, 212
confusion, 159
conjugated linoleic acid (CLA), 134–35, 150 (table)
connective tissue, 78
convulsions, 160
coping skills, 209–10
corn syrup, 107
corosolic acid, 141, 150 (table)
counselors, professional, 210–11, 214
cow's milk, and diabetes risk, 8
Coxsackie viruses, 7
crankiness, 212
creatine, 118, 132
creatinine, 118
cross-country skiing, 73
cryptoxanthin, 114
cuts and bruises, slow-to-heal, 4 (table)

Daily Reference Intake (DRI), 66
daily requirements, calculating, 82–86
dairy products, 63, 64
death, causes of, in the United States, 3
dehydration, 91, 167
dental exam, scheduling, 51 (table)
dental surgery, 37 (table)
dentist, 42
depression, clinical, 71, 76, 211–15
dermatologist, 42
desaturase, 136
desserts, 62

dextrose, 107
DiaBeta, 194, 196 (table)
diabetes
  description and types of, 4–20
  diagnosis of, xiii, 24–27
  early warning signs, 4 (table), 44
  learning about, 20–23
  life-threatening complications of, 28–37
  number of people who have it, 3
  risk factors for, 7–16
  six steps to control, xvi, 81
  See also type 1 diabetes; type 2 diabetes
diabetes care plan, 46–48
Diabetes Complications and Control Trial, 154
Diabetes Forecast, 22
  Buyer's Guide, 191
diabetic foods (marketed as such), 71
Diabinese, 194, 196 (table), 198
diagnostic tests, 25–27
diarrhea, 34
diet, 81–111
  easing into changes in, 81–90
dietary supplements, 42, 112–52
  designing a program of, 146–52, 149–150 (table)
dietitian, registered, 41
digestion, 34, 63, 90
  poor, 33
distal symmetric neuropathy, 33, 54
dizziness, 159, 165
doctors
  finding and choosing, 38–40
  follow-up visits to, schedule of, 48–50
  initial visit to, what to expect, 45–48
  list of questions for, 21
drowsiness, 4 (table)
drug exposure, and diabetes risk, 9
duration (insulin characteristic), 56

eating out, gauging portions while, 97
eggs, 63
Elavil, 213
electrocardiogram (EKG), 46
eleuthero, 144
emergencies, 158–62
emotional health, maintaining, 222–23
end-stage renal disease, 33
energy, low, 112
enzymes, 9
  fat-burning, 74
Eskimos, 137
essential fatty acids, 64, 136, 151
estrogen, 107
evening primrose oil, 136–37, 150 (table)
exchange lists, 91–94, 98 (table)
exercise, 10, 14, 18, 72–78, 151, 163–86
  aerobic, 73–76, 169–74
  benefits of, 72–77, 108–9, 163
  choice of, 52–53, 169–70, 174, 183–184 (table)
  duration, frequency, and intensity of, 170–77
  metabolism problems during, 164–69
  safety considerations, 164–69
  sticking to a routine of, 181–82
  strength training, 76–78
exercise physiologist, 41
exercise plan, preparticipation evaluation for setting up, 50–55
exercising heart rate, 171–72
extremities
  circulation of, 52
  pain in the, 33
eye diseases and damage, 73
  diabetes causing, 30–32
  and exercise choice, 53
eye exam, dilated, schedule of, 51 (table)

fainting, 165
family history, 6
family relationships, and health, 217–19
family therapists, 42
fasting plasma glucose test, 12, 25
fat, body, 105, 135
   exercise to control, 74, 77
fat, dietary, 63–65
   beneficial, 134–38
   daily need for, how to calculate, 85–86
   eating less of, 86–87
   saturated or unsaturated, 64–65
"fat baby," 19
fatigue, 4 (table), 159, 212
fats, sweets, and alcohol food group, 97
fatty acids, 14, 15, 70, 74
fear, overcoming, 216–17
feeling, loss of, 34
feet, 35, 52, 53, 120
   cold, 52
   poor circulation of, 29
fenugreek, 141–42, 150 (table)
fever, 161
fiber, 88, 90 (table), 106
finger-stick test, 155–56
fish, 63, 64, 65
fish oil, 137–38, 150 (table)
focal neuropathy, 33–34, 54
food
   combinations of, 100
   fat-forming, 105
   fiber-rich, 90 (table)
   "forbidden," 66–71
   glycemic index of, 100–103
   high-fiber, 88–89, 106
   natural, 88–89
   variety of, 87–88
   See also diet
food pyramid for diabetics, 95–97, 99 (table)

foot exam, scheduling, 51 (table)
footwear, 37 (table), 53, 54, 164
forgetfulness, 212
free radicals
   controlling, 113
   and diabetes risk, 8–9, 16
fructose, 62
fruit, 62
fruit food group, 96

galactose, 62
gamma-carotene, 114
gamma-linolenic acid (GLA), 136, 151
gangrene, 29, 52
garlic, 142–43, 150 (table)
Gatorade, 168
general physical exam, 51 (table)
German measles, 7
gestational diabetes, 12, 18–20, 124
   testing for, 26–27
ginseng, 143–44, 150 (table)
Glargine, 59 (table)
glaucoma, 32
glimepiride, 194
glipizide, 194
globin, 76
glossary of medical terms, 225–32
glucokinase, 123
Glucophage, 126, 138, 195–97, 198, 199, 200, 202
glucose
   in blood. *See* blood sugar
   physiology of, 4–6, 62, 76, 94, 123
   slow release of, foods that promote, 100–103
glucose intolerance, 15
glucose meter, 155–56
glucose tablets or gels, 159
glucose transporter, 11
Glucotrol, 194–95, 196 (table), 199

Glucotrol XL, 194, 196 (table)
Glucovance, 202–3
GlucoWatch, 156
glutathione, 120
glyburide, 143, 194, 202
glycation, 48–49, 76, 115–16, 118, 124
    reduction of, 121
glycemic index, 100–103, 102–103 (table)
glycogen, 70
glycohemoglobin (GHb) test, 48–49, 208
    scheduling, 51 (table)
glycosuria, 128
Glynase, 194, 196 (table)
Glyset, 198
grains, beans, starchy vegetable food group, 95–96
gum infection, 4 (table), 35, 37 (table)
gymnema silvestre, 144–45, 150 (table)
gymnemic acid, 145

hands, 120
HbA1C and HbA1 tests, 49
Head, Kathleen, 148
headache, 159, 160
health
    family relationships and, 217–19
    spiritual faith and, 219–21
health care professionals, finding, 40–43
Health Professionals Follow-Up, 99
heart, 74
heart disease, 70–71, 73, 113
    diabetes causing, 28–29
    exercise to combat, 74–75, 183 (table)
    prevention of, 36, 36 (table), 119
    treatment of, 36, 36 (table)
heart rate, 54, 75
    during exercise, 171–72
heartbeat, 34
    irregular, 122
    rapid, 159

hemoglobin, 115–16
herbs, 42, 147, 150 (table)
herbs, medicinal, 138–46
heredity, and diabetes risk, 7, 12–13
high blood pressure (hypertension), 15, 73, 127, 129–30
    diabetes causing, 29–30
    diet to reduce, 108–9
    exercise to reduce, 75, 108–9
    prevention and treatment of, 36 (table)
hiking, 170
Hispanics, 13, 19
HMOs, 43
homocysteine, 124
Huemer, Richard P., 205
human insulin, 56
hunger, 159
    unexplained, 4 (table)
hydrogenation, 65
hydroxyl radical, 120
hyperglycemia, 5, 113, 160–62, 166, 208, 211
hyperlipdemia, 15
hypertension, 29–30. *See* high blood pressure
hypnotherapy, 42
hypoglycemia, 70, 158–60, 166, 208, 211
hypoglycemic reaction, 159–60

ice cream, 100
identification bracelet, 164
immune system, 6, 7, 34
impaired glucose tolerance (IGT), 12, 26
impotence, 33, 34
inactivity, and diabetes risk, 14–15
infections, 4 (table), 52
    diabetes causing, 34–35
    prevention and treatment of, 37 (table)
infuser, 190
inhaled insulin, 191

injection aids, 191
injection of insulin
　techniques, 188–93
　where to inject, 192
injector, insulin, 190
inositol, 125
insomnia, 212
insulin, natural
　chromium's effect on, 127
　deficiency of, 5
　exercise helping use of, 77
　physiology of, 4–6
insulin, supplemental (self-administered),
　　9–10, 55–57, 188–93, 195, 203
　frequency of use of, 192–93
　hypoglycemic reaction from, 159–60
　injection of, 188–93
　reducing amount needed, 72, 105
　storing, 193 (table)
　types and basic characteristics of,
　　55–57, 58–59 (table)
insulin-dependent diabetes, 5
insulin pump, 189–90
insulin reaction (hypoglycemic), 159–60
insulin resistance, 5, 11, 30
insurance plans, 43
interleukin-6, 220
intermittent claudification, 29, 52
irritability, 4 (table), 212
islets of Langerbans, 6

jaw, discomfort in, 165
jogging, 52, 54, 73
joints, 78
Joslin Diabetes Centers, 22
juvenile-onset diabetes, 5

Kelly, Gregory S., N.D., 134
ketoacidosis, 160–62, 167
ketones, 46, 161, 166

kidney dialysis, 33
kidney disease. *See* nephropathy
kidneys, 30, 32
　transplants, 33

laboratory tests, 46
lactic acidosis, 197
lactose, 62, 107
Lantus, 59 (table)
laser treatment, 36 (table)
Latinos, 12
legs, 35, 52
　pain and cramps, 52
　poor circulation in, 29
legumes, 63
Lente, 58 (table)
lifting weights, 53, 73
ligaments, 78
linoleic acid, 64, 134, 136
linolenic acid, 64
lipid peroxidation, 117, 131
lipid profile test, scheduling, 51 (table)
lipoprotein lipase, 135
liquid insulin, 191
lispro, 58 (table)
liver, 59
liver glycogen, 62
love, and health, 217–19
lutein, 114
lycopene, 114

macrosomia (fat baby), 19
macular edema, 32
magnesium, 108, 128–29, 149 (table)
maltitol, 68
maltodextrin, 107
maltose, 107
mannitol, 68
margarines, 65
marker, 118

massage, 42
meals
　mixed, 100
　multiple throughout the day, 89–90
　planning, 10, 17, 91–97, 93 (table), 98–99 (table)
　preparation tips, 104
　sample daily menu, 92 (table)
meat, 63, 64
meat and others food group, 96
Med-Alert, 164
medical care, getting the best, 205–6
medical history, 45
medical tests, 44–54
　scheduling, 51 (table)
medical waste, disposing of, 189
medication, 55–59, 187–206
　getting off, 163
　reducing amount needed, 72, 88
meditation, 151
meglitinides, 200–201
memory problems, 212
mental health, exercise as promoting, 76
mental health therapist, 42
metabolism, 74, 77
　exercise and, 164–69
　rate of, 90
metformin, 126, 138, 195, 202, 203
methionione, 124
methylhydroxy chalcone polymer (MHCP), 140
Michelis, Mary Kay, 205
Micronase, 194, 196 (table), 198, 199
milk food group, 96
milk thistle, 145–46, 150 (table)
minerals, 65–66, 147, 149 (table)
　supplementary, 125–31
mitochondria, 122, 133
monoamine oxidase (MAO) inhibitors, 216

mood swings, 212
mouth, 35
　dry, 161
mumps, 7
muscle cells, 14–15, 77
muscle glycogen, 62
muscle tone, exercise and, 78
muscles, 72, 75, 76
　breakdown of, instead of glucose, 6
　lean, 77
muscular coordination, 34
muscular tension, 76

Nardil, 217
National Committee of Quality Assurance (NCQA), 43
National Institute of Diabetes and Digestive and Kidney Diseases, 22
natural remedies. *See* dietary supplements
nausea, 165
neck, discomfort in, 165
neomyrtillin, 139
nephrons, 32
nephropathy (kidney disease), 69, 73, 84, 113
　diabetes causing, 32–33
　and exercise choice, 53, 183 (table)
　prevention of, 36 (table), 118–19
　treatment of, 36 (table)
nerves
　damage to, 73
　loss of tissue, 54
nervousness, 159
neuropathy (nervous system disease), 124, 125
　diabetes causing, 33–34
　and exercise choice, 54, 184 (table)
　prevention and treatment of, 37 (table)

repair of, from dietary supplements, 120–21
types of, 33–34
niacinamide, 124
nicotine, 17
non-insulin-dependent diabetes, 10
non-weight-bearing activity, 54
NPH, 58 (table)
numbness, 4 (table), 29, 33, 54
Nurses' Health Study, 99
nutrients, 89
nutrition, 14, 61–71. *See also* diet
nutritional drinks, 132

obesity, 12, 30
   and diabetes risk, 13–14
   exercise to combat, 74
   See also fat, body; weight loss
oils, cooking, 64–65
omega-3 fatty acids, 65, 137–38
omega-6 fatty acids, 65
on-line support groups, 215
onset (insulin characteristic), 56
ophthalmologist, 41
oral diabetes medications, 57–60, 187, 193–204
oral glucose tolerance test, 12, 25–26
oral hypoglycemic agents, 57
Orinase, 194, 196 (table)
osteoporosis, 78
oxidative stress, 113
oxygen-processing capacity, 74

Pacific Islanders, 12, 13, 19
pain, 34, 52, 165
Pamelor, 213
pancreas, 4–5, 6, 9, 57, 59
pantethine, 125
pantothenic acid, 125
Parnate, 217

Paxil, 213
peak time (insulin characteristic), 56
pen injector, 190
pentamidine, 9
peroxides, 117, 131
pharmacist, 42
D-phenylalanine derivatives, 201
phobias, overcoming, 216–17
photocoagulation, 36 (table)
physical examination, 46
Pima Indians, 137
pioglitazone hydrocloride, 199
platelets, 75
   aggregation of, 204
pleasure, loss of interest in, 212
Pleasure Break, 223
podiatrist, 41
polio, 7
polyols, 151
positive living, 207, 221–23
potassium, 108, 129–30, 149 (table)
Prandin, 200–201
Precose, 198
pregnancy, 60, 194
   and diabetes risk, 18–20
premixed insulin, 57
processed foods, 62, 65, 69, 89, 105, 107
prostaglandins, 136
protein food, 63
   daily need for, how to calculate, 84–85
   restricted diet of, 84
proteins, body, glycation of, 124
Provider Recognition Program, 39
Prozac, 213
psychiatrists, 42
psychologists, clinical, 42
pulse, 52
pump, insulin, 189–90
Pyriminil, 9

quercetin, 151

racial background, and diabetes risk, 7
racquet sports, 53, 170
random plasma glucose test, 25
rating of perceived exertion (RPE), 172–73
reaction-products, 159
receptors (cell), 11
recommended daily allowance (RDA), 66
red blood cells, 124
   glycated, 48–49, 115–16
relationships with family and friends, and health, 217–19
relaxation techniques, 42–43
resources for diabetes management (books, websites, etc.), 233–41
respiration, 34
respiratory tract infections, 35
restaurants, eating at, 97
retina, 30
retinopathy, 113
   diabetes causing, 30–32
   and exercise choice, 53, 183 (table)
   nonproliferative and proliferative, 31–32
   prevention of, 36 (table), 118–19
   treatment of, 36 (table)
rewarding yourself, 182
risk factors
   for type 1 diabetes, 6–9
   for type 2 diabetes, 12–17
rosiglitazone maleate, 199
rowing, 54
rubber band exercise equipment, 73
"runner's high," 76
running, 53, 73

saccharin, 67
sadness, persistent, 212

Saint-John's-wort, 214
salt, 30, 68, 108
saponins, 142
satiation, 106
Schwambach, Judith, 222
screening tests, 24–25
sedentary lifestyle, 12, 14
selective serotonin reuptake inhibitors (SSRIs), 213
self-esteem, lack of, 212
self-monitoring of blood glucose (SMBG), 153–62
   recording your results, 157–58
   types of tests, 155–56
   when to test, 157
Serax, 216
serum creatinine, 46
sex interest, 212
shakiness, 159
side effects, 194, 195–97, 199–200, 201, 202–3
silymarin, 145
skin, 35
   dry, itchy, 160, 161
   infection, 4 (table)
sleepiness, 161
smoking, and diabetes risk, 17
snack foods, 15
snacks (between meals), 89
social workers, 42
sodium, 30, 68–69
sorbitol, 68, 116
sores, 54
spiritual faith, and health, 219–21
sports, 100
   diabetes and, 179–80
sports drinks and bars, 132, 168
Starlix, 201
stationary cycling, 53, 170
step aerobics, 54

stevia, 67–68
steviocide, 67
steviol, 67
stomach muscles, 34
stomach pains, 161
strength (insulin characteristic), 56
strength training, 53, 73, 76–78
  benefits of, 76–78
  intensity of, 175
  sets per exercise, 176
  setting up a program of, 174–79, 178–180 (table)
stress, 76, 151
  managing, 10, 207, 208–11
stress hormones, 30
stroke, 73
  diabetes causing, 29
  prevention and treatment of, 36 (table)
subcutaneous injections, 189
sucrose, 62, 107
sugar (food), 22, 91, 99, 107
  in diet, limiting, 62, 67–68
sugar alcohols, 68
suicide, thoughts of, 212
sulfonylureas, 194–95, 196 (table), 202, 203
supplementary minerals, 125–31
support groups, 214–15
  on-line, 215
sweeteners, artificial, 67–68
swimming, 53, 54, 73, 170
Syndrome X, 12, 15
  and diabetes risk, 15–16
syringe, 189
systematic desensitization, 217
systolic blood pressure, 53

T cells, 6
talk test (of exercise intensity), 173–74
L-taurine, 133–34, 150 (table)

teenagers, diabetes in, 16
teeth, 126
tendons, 78
tension, 212
test kits, 161–62
thermogenesis, 90
thiazolidinediones, 199–200
thirst, excessive or extreme, 4 (table), 33, 160, 161
thyroid-stimulating hormone, 46
tingling, 4 (table), 33
toes, 53
tolbutamide, 194
trans-fatty acids, 65
Tranxene, 216
treadmill exercise, 54, 73
treadmill stress test, 46
tricyclic antidepressants (TCAs), 213
triglycerides, 28, 63, 71, 137–38
  reducing level of, 77, 107–8
  risk levels, 46, 47 (table)
trigonelline, 142
tropical oils, 64
twin studies, 12–13
type 1 diabetes, 5–10, 106, 157, 158
  risk factors for, 6–9
  treatments for, 9–10
type 2 diabetes, 10–18, 99, 105, 107, 135, 137, 157, 158, 202, 208
  risk factors for, 12–17
  treatments for, 17–18, 57–60, 187, 193–204

ulcers, 29
ultralente, 58 (table)
unconsciousness, 159–60
unhappiness, 212
United States Department of Agriculture, 95
urinary tract infection, 34, 35

urination, frequent, 4 (table), 33, 160, 161
urine, 128
urine protein level, 46
urine tests, 161–62
   scheduling, 51 (table)

vaginal infections, 35, 37 (table)
Valium, 216
vanadium, 130, 150 (table)
vanadyl sulfate, 130
vegetable food group, 62, 96
very-low-density lipoprotein (VLDL), 64
virus attack, and diabetes risk, 7
vision
   blurry, 4 (table), 160, 161
   problems with, after exercise, 165
vitamin A, 114
vitamin B_1 (thiamine), 123–24
vitamin B_3 (niacin), 124
vitamin B_6 (pyroxidine), 124
vitamin B_{12} (cobalamin), 124–25, 126
vitamin C, 115–16, 149 (table), 151

vitamin E, 117–19, 138, 149 (table), 151
vitamins, 65–66
volleyball, 170
vomiting, 34, 161

walking, 53, 54, 73, 169
water, drinking, 91, 165
water exercise, 53
weakness, 161
weight loss, 17, 33, 74, 108
   diet and exercise to achieve, 105–7
   unusual, 4 (table)
weight-training machines, 73
weight lifting, 53, 73
whites, 7

Xanax, 216
xylitol, 68

yoga, 42, 151

zinc, 131, 150 (table)
Zoloft, 213